D1105157

Colposcopy

Text and Atlas

Louis Burke, MD
Associate Professor, Obstetrics and Gynecology
Harvard Medical School
Associate Director and Obstetrician-Gynecologist-in-Chief-Emeritus
Director, Colposcopy and Laser Clinic
Department of Obstetrics and Gynecology
Beth Israel Hospital
Boston, Massachusetts

Donald A. Antonioli, MD
Associate Professor, Pathology
Harvard Medical School
Associate Chief, Department of Pathology
Beth Israel Hospital
Boston, Massachusetts

Barbara S. Ducatman, MD
Assistant Professor, Pathology
Harvard Medical School
Medical Director, Cytopathology Laboratory
Beth Israel Hospital
Boston, Massachusetts

With a Foreword by

Adolf Stafl, MD, PhD
Professor
Department of Obstetrics and Gynecology
Medical College of Wisconsin
Milwaukee, Wisconsin

APPLETON & LANGE
Norwalk, Connecticut/San Mateo, California

0-8385-0523-6

Notice: Our knowledge in clinical sciences is constantly changing. As new
information becomes available, changes in treatment and in the use of drugs
become necessary. The authors and the publisher of this volume have taken
care to make certain that the doses of drugs and schedules of treatment are
correct and compatible with the standards generally accepted at the time of
publication. The reader is advised to consult carefully the instruction
and information material included in the package insert of each drug or
therapeutic agent before administration. This advice is especially
important when using new or infrequently used drugs.

Copyright © 1991 by Appleton & Lange
A Publishing Division of Prentice Hall

All rights reserved. This book, or any parts thereof, may not be used or
reproduced in any manner without written permission. For information,
address Appleton & Lange, 25 Van Zant Street, East Norwalk, Connecticut 06855.

91 92 93 94 95 / 10 9 8 7 6 5 4 3 2 1

Prentice Hall International (UK) Limited, *London*
Prentice Hall of Australia Pty. Limited, *Sydney*
Prentice Hall Canada, Inc., *Toronto*
Prentice Hall Hispanoamericana, S.A., *Mexico*
Prentice Hall of India Private Limited, *New Delhi*
Prentice Hall of Japan, Inc., *Tokyo*
Simon & Schuster Asia Pte. Ltd., *Singapore*
Editora Prentice Hall do Brasil Ltda., *Rio de Janeiro*
Prentice Hall, *Englewood Cliffs, New Jersey*

Library of Congress Cataloging-in-Publication Data

Burke, Louis, 1920–
    Basic and advanced colposcopy / Louis Burke, Donald A. Antonioli,
Barbara S. Ducatman.
        p.   cm.
    ISBN 0-8385-0523-6
    1. Colposcopy.   I. Antonioli, Donald A.   II. Ducatman, Barbara S.
III. Title.
    [DNLM: 1. Cervix Diseases—diagnosis. 2. Colposcopy. 3. Vaginal
Diseases—diagnosis. 4. Vulvar Diseases—diagnosis. WP 250 B959b]
RG107.5.C6B86   1990
618.1 '4—dc20
DNLM/DLC
for Library of Congress   90–1001
                                                                  CIP

Editor: R. Craig Percy
Designer: Janice Barsevich

PRINTED IN THE UNITED STATES OF AMERICA

*Dedicated to Dorothy Burke, Anna Antonioli, and Alan Ducatman.
Patience, empathy, and understanding made this book possible.*

Contents

A color plate section follows page 214.

Foreword

Colposcopy is today recognized as an inseparable part of the evaluation of patients with abnormal cytology. Twenty years ago the usual procedure to evaluate patients with suspicious cytology was conization. In addition, the management of preinvasive cervical disease was more radical, and the only definitive treatment of a carcinoma in situ of the cervix was hysterectomy with a wide vaginal cuff. The introduction of colposcopy significantly changed this practice. It was proven that colposcopy can identify the most suspicious area on the cervix that can be sampled in directed biopsy. Thus, in most cases, the necessity for conization can be avoided. Expert colposcopic evaluation can rule out the presence of invasive carcinoma, allowing preinvasive cervical lesions to be treated conservatively by local destruction alone.

The colposcope was first developed by Hinselmann in 1925, and colposcopy was used for years in Europe and in South America mainly as a competitive method to cytology. In the late 1960s and early 1970s several physicians in the United States recognized that the main role of colposcopy is not cervical cancer screening but rather evaluation of patients with abnormal cytology. From this point the interest in colposcopy in the United States grew. With the use of colposcopy the frequency of conization dropped significantly and the need for conization during pregnancy almost disappeared. Colposcopy also significantly changed the management of cervical intraepithelial neoplasia. Cryosurgery and laser therapy developed because colposcopy provided a more precise diagnosis.

One of the pioneers of colposcopy in the United States was Dr. Louis Burke, who was associated with the early development of colposcopy in this country and made valuable contributions himself. Many colposcopy teaching courses were organized by him, and hundreds of gynecologists were introduced to colposcopy through his teaching efforts. He always stressed that colposcopy cannot be learned only by looking through the instrument, but at the pathologist's bench as well. Every colposcopic lesson has a pathologic counterpart, and the proper clinical interpretation of the significance of these lesions must be done by physicians with experience in both colposcopy and pathology. Dr. Burke was also very active in the American Society of Colposcopy and Cervical Pathology. He spent many years on the Board of Directors, and from 1984 to 1986 was president of the society.

Dr. Burke is writing from his personal experiences. His long-term teaching practice in colposcopy is condensed in this book. The importance of correlation between colposcopy, histology, and cytology is stressed, and the many colposcopy pictures are supplemented with corresponding histologic findings. This book provides both basic information for the beginning colposcopist as well as practical guidelines for a more experienced colposcopist. Dr. Burke also addresses new horizons of colposcopy such as cervicography. As one of the first users of this method, he presents representative cervicography photographs and explains the place of cervicography in gynecology.

The lifelong mission of Dr. Burke has been colposcopy teaching. There is no doubt that this book will be an excellent guide to its users in their colposcopic practice.

Adolf Stafl, MD, PhD

Preface

The contents of this book are based on our experience in teaching colposcopy at many basic and advanced courses sponsored by the Harvard Medical School Department of Continuing Medical Education and the American Society for Colposcopy and Cervical Pathology. It quickly became apparent to us that a knowledge of the morphologic basis of colposcopy is necessary for both the neophyte and the experienced colposcopist. We have attempted to crystallize this clinicopathologic approach in analyzing the numerous gynecologic problems for which colposcopy is indicated.

The efficacy of colposcopy for the detection and diagnosis of preinvasive and invasive neoplastic lesions of the cervix is now generally accepted. Renewed interest in the method has occurred because of the increase in similar lesions involving the vagina, vulva, and, to a lesser extent, the perianal region. The use of colposcopy to evaluate these structures has markedly widened the scope of the technique.

In addition, in the past decade we have seen a marked increase in the number of cases of sexually transmitted diseases, in particular those related to human papilloma virus infection. Concurrently, the mean age of occurrence for precursor lesions of the cervix, vagina, and vulva has decreased. As a result, new methods of treatment that do not interfere with childbearing and coital function have had to be devised. Developed over the past 10 years, laser surgery, which fulfills the criterion of being a nonmutilating therapy, requires the use of colposcopy for optimal benefit. Expertise in colposcopy is necessary to triage patients with these various lesions prior to laser surgery.

The organization of this book is a sequential presentation of the histologic, cytologic, and colposcopic features of the various diseases of the lower female genital tract. The physiologic bases for the observed colposcopic changes are reviewed. Correlation of the morphologic changes with the colposcopic findings is stressed. We have also included information on other techniques, such as cervicography and the use of salicylic acid, that may be useful to augment the traditional modalities of the colposcopic evaluation.

This volume should be a useful clinical reference for medical students, house officers, and practicing health care personnel, especially gynecologists. We have attempted to make this book of value to the pathologist interested in the diseases of the cervix, vagina, and vulva.

Preparation of this text was supported by a grant from Carl Zeiss, Inc., Thornwood, New York. The authors and publisher extend their thanks to them.

Louis Burke, MD
Donald A. Antonioli, MD
Barbara S. Ducatman, MD

Chapter 1 | Tissue Basis of Colposcopy

HISTORY OF COLPOSCOPY

The cervix and vagina first became accessible for direct inspection as a result of the invention of the vaginal speculum by Recamier in 1818. With access to the cervix, investigators began to elucidate the natural history of cervical cancer. In 1925, Hinselmann made his significant contribution to this study by inventing the colposcope, an instrument based on his concept that the primary focus of cervical cancer was a minute ulceration that could not be appreciated by gross inspection with the naked eye (Figure 1–1). The colposcope provided magnification and high intensity illumination to delineate this early lesion. In this way, the new field of colposcopy was invented.

Colposcopy, which may be defined as the examination of epithelial surfaces with a low-power microscope and a strong light, initially was not widely accepted in English speaking countries and, indeed, was derided. There were several reasons for this delay in acceptance. All of the early reports were in German, which introduced a language barrier to the understanding of colposcopy. Terminology was based on visual impressions that could not be clearly related to the histology or pathophysiology of tumor development and growth. A third reason was that colposcopy and cytology, the latter having been developed at about the same time by Papanicolaou, were initially construed as competitive rather than as complimentary techniques for cervical cancer detection.

In the 1960s, however, colposcopy began to enjoy a growing popularity in English speaking countries, based on an improved understanding of the morphologic basis for the colposcopic images and the recognition of the complimentary roles of cytology and colposcopy in the detection of neoplasia.

In the modern practice of gynecology, colposcopy has become an integral part of the gynecologic examination. Colposcopy, however, cannot be done in a vacuum; rather, it must be performed in concert with cytology and tissue sampling. In addition, we believe that colposcopy is best learned at the pathologist's bench. Every colposcopic image is the counterpart of a specific tissue pattern, which in turn is determined by the interplay of the surface epithelium with its connective tissue stroma. The colposcopic image is produced by illuminating both the surface epithelium and the underlying stroma; it is a reflection of epithelial cell number, organization, and morphology, and it is also influenced by the vascular arrangement of the adjacent stroma. Because various combinations of epithelial and stromal abnormalities produce identifiable colposcopic images, both normal and abnormal epithelia assume colposcopic appearances almost as characteristic as those seen on histologic examination.

1

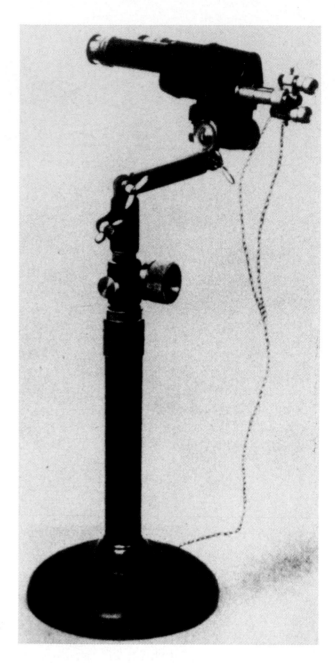

Figure 1-1 Hinselmann's original colposcope.

BASIC COLPOSCOPIC IMAGES

The Normal Epithelium

If a strip of normal stratified squamous epithelium is interposed between the strong light of the colposcope and the observing eye, the image formed is the result of the light traversing the superficial glycogenated cells and the basal layers of the squamous mucosa to reach the underlying lamina propria (Figure 1-2, Color Plate 1). Thus, the reflected image will be influenced by the presence of intravascular red blood cells and will be in the red color range. The thinner the epithelium, the redder the image; the thicker the epithelium, the paler the red hue. Normally, no blood vessels extend into the epithelium except for those in the stromal papillae confined to the basal zone of the epithelium (*see* Chapter 2). The epithelial surface will be either flat or slightly undulating.

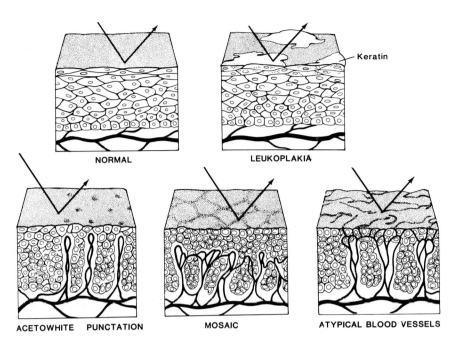

Figure 1-2. Tissue basis of colposcopy.

Leukoplakia and Keratosis

If the squamous epithelium has plaques of keratin on its surface, the light cannot traverse the epithelial cells and reach the blood in the vessels in the lamina propria. Thus, rather than being red, the visual image is a white plaque (Figure 1–3). Keratin thickens the surface; the plaque is, therefore, raised above the adjacent nonkeratotic mucosa and will have an elevated, well-defined margin. These raised white plaques are called *leukoplakia* or *keratosis*. By definition, they can be identified without colposcopy by use of a good light and careful visual inspection. Also, the recognition of leukoplakia is not dependent on the topical application of solutions such as acetic acid.

If the squamous mucosa consists of immature cells, the colposcopic image will differ from the normal. The cells of immature mucosa contain increased amounts of nuclear DNA, have denser than normal cytoplasm, and increased nuclear:cytoplasmic ratios. Consequently, the ability of light to pass through the epithelium will be diminished, and the result will be an opacity or whiteness of the surface in the abnormal area (Figure 1–4). This whiteness can be enhanced by washing the surface of the epithelium with dilute acetic acid.

Aceto-White Epithelium

The exact mechanism whereby acetic acid causes a color change was never elucidated by Hinselmann, and the precise basis for the change remains obscure today. We believe the white image is primarily due to an osmolar change: acetic acid causes water to leave the cell, after which the cell membrane collapses around the abnormal and large nucleus. Thus, light transmission is interrupted, and the lesion appears white. Over time, as the acetic acid dissipates from the tissue, the osmolar change is reversed, water returns to the cell, and the whiteness fades. The intensity of the whiteness, its speed of appearance, its duration, and the rapidity of its disappearance are all related to the number of immature cells. The greater the number of such cells, the more intense the whiteness, the faster the change will develop, and the longer its duration. This type of visual image is called *aceto-white epithelium*. Unlike leukoplakia, it can be seen only with magnifica-

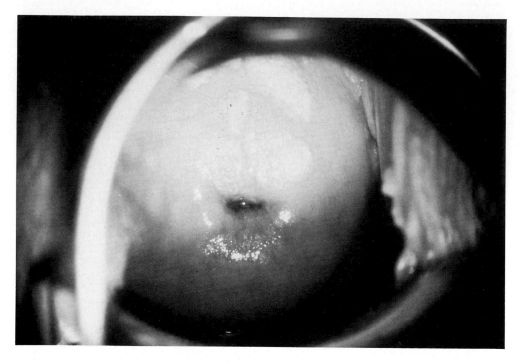

Figure 1-3. Cervix prior to the application of acetic acid, with areas of leukoplakia. Elevated, well defined lesions are obvious on the anterior cervical lip. Histologically, prominent keratinization is present.

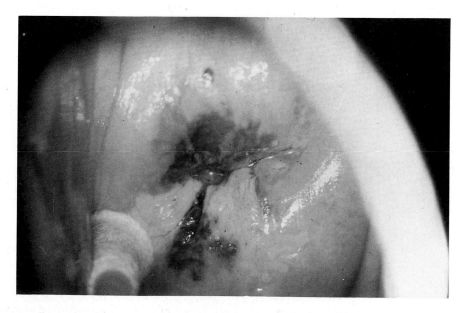

Figure 1-4. Cervix after the application of 3% acetic acid. Two sharply delineated aceto-white areas are obvious at four to six and seven to eight o'clock.

tion by means of colposcopy. Its presence is transient, but it can be renewed by the reapplication of acetic acid.

Punctation and Mosaic Patterns

If we now combine the same block of immature cells with a change in vascularity in which the blood vessels, rather than being confined to the lamina propria, extend to the surface of the epithelium, a distinctive pattern called *punctation* will be identified. Prior to the application of acetic acid, the tips of the vessels will be seen in the epithelium as red dots. After the application of acetic acid, these red tips are seen perforating the aceto-white epithelium. If the vasculature does not reach the surface, however, but rather extends only partially through the epithelium, it forms a basketlike network around the blocks of immature cells and a distinctive colposcopic image called a *mosaic* structure ensues. After the application of acetic acid, the top of the basketlike arrangement of vessels that surrounds the abnormal blocks of cells is identified as a red line (Figure 1–5). The appearance is reminiscent of tiles on a floor and, thus, the term "mosaicism" is used to describe the image.

Atypical Blood Vessels

If new capillaries are formed, they usually have a distinctive appearance (ie vessels tend to be parallel to the surface and arborization does not occur) (Figure 1–6, Color Plate 2). This development is the fifth colposcopic image and is termed *atypical blood vessels* and will be more fully discussed in Chapter 5.

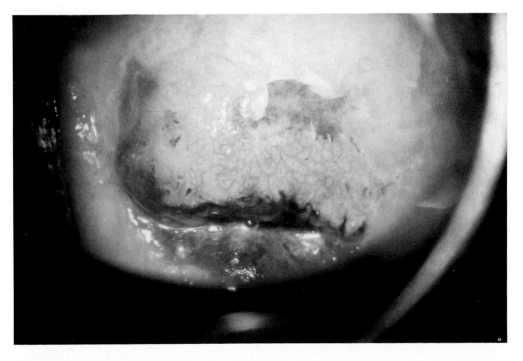

Figure 1–5. Colpophotograph of cervix after 3% acetic acid. Mosaicism is obvious on the anterior lip of the cervix.

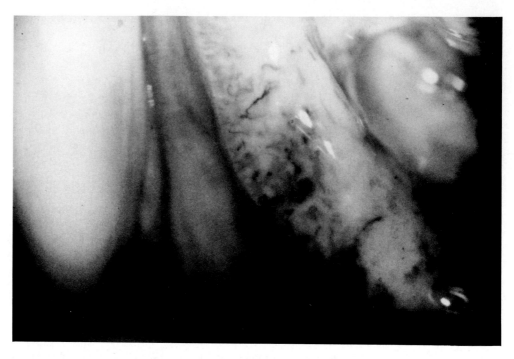

Figure 1-6. Atypical blood vessels at the edge of an invasive squamous cell carcinoma of the cervix. Note the nondividing abnormal vessel that is parallel to the surface and very superficial.

SUMMARY

The five images of leukoplakia, aceto-white epithelium, punctation, mosaic pattern, and atypical blood vessels are the basic descriptive vocabulary of the colposcopic method. Any process that increases keratin production, increases cellular division, increases vascular changes, and produces new blood vessels can cause any of these abnormal images. Thus, metaplasia, infection, inflammation, regeneration, repair and, most importantly, neoplasia can produce the changes. As we shall subsequently see, the changes of neoplasia can for the most part be distinguished from the less important changes causing these various colposcopic appearances.

Because the epithelial surface of any accessible organ is amenable to investigation, the cervix, vagina, vulva, anus, oral cavity, and penis are areas that lend themselves to examination by colposcopy. In this book, we attempt to summarize the value of colposcopy in modern gynecology through an understanding of cytology and histopathology, as well as the colposcopic images of various disease states. Our goal is to aid the gynecologist in evaluation and treatment of his or her patients.

Chapter 2 | Instrumentation and Biopsy Techniques

INSTRUMENTATION

All colposcopes basically consist of the following components:

1. Optics, eyepieces, and filters.
2. Light source.
3. Stand.
4. Ancillary equipment.

Colposcopes contain a stereoscopic binocular microscope with low-magnification objective lenses, usually $10 \times$ to $40 \times$. The instrument is equipped with a centered illuminating device and can be placed on a variety of stands.

Optics

Colposcopes fall into two general categories: (1) those containing a single objective lens with a fixed focal distance and whose magnification can only be altered by changing the power of the eyepieces (Figure 2–1); and (2) instruments with a single objective lens but with multiple magnifiers built into the body of the microscope (Figure 2–2). The objective lens influences the working distance between the instrument and the field of examination. The best focal length, or working distance, for a colposcope is between 250 and 300 mm, and most colposcopes are fitted with lenses to provide focal lengths within this range.

The biopsy instruments of 20 to 25 cm in length, commonly used a decade ago, are usually awkward to manipulate; therefore, the more modern biopsy instruments, that are less than 20 cm in length, are preferable. If long instruments are used, colposcopes with an objective lens of 300 mm are preferred. Lenses with short focal lengths of 100 to 200 mm are best for detailed study of lesions and for obtaining photographs. The usual colposcope contains a 250 mm lens that will accommodate the modern instruments.

The method of moving the focusing element varies among colposcopes: some have very fine adjustment knobs whereas others involve coarse movement of the head of the scope. Zoom capability with continuous focusing is offered by some manufacturers. With 200 to 250 mm objectives and a $10 \times$ eyepiece, the diameter of the visualized field ranges from 20 to 23 mm. Increasing the focal length of the objective lens at any given magnification will increase the diameter of the visualized field.

Colposcopes with multiple magnification capabilities are equipped with a knob with varied settings (*see* Figure 2–2). Refocusing is usually not necessary when the knob is turned to change magnification. At any given setting, the magnification is further altered

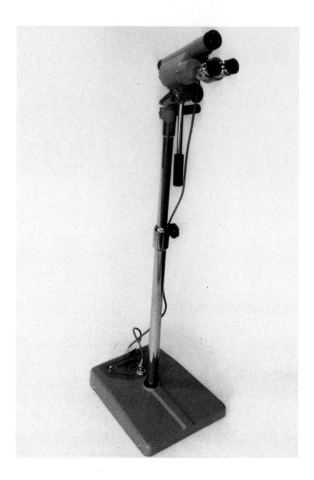

Figure 2-1. Fixed focus colposcope on broad foot base.

by the objective lens and the strength of the eyepieces. Magnification of 10× to 16× is satisfactory for routine examinations of the mucous membranes. Use of lower magnifications of 5× to 10× offers the advantages of easy, rapid screening and panoramic viewing, especially helpful features in vaginal and vulvar colposcopy. Magnification of 20× to 40× is needed for detailed evaluation of blood vessels. High magnification, however, decreases the field of vision, the depth of focus, and causes the loss of architectural orientation (Table 2–1).

Eyepieces

Many colposcope manufacturers give the examiner a choice of eyepieces with magnifications varying from 10× to 20×. The eyepieces may have independent focusing elements adaptable to the individual's own eyesight. Elements to allow adjustment for an individual's interocular distance are part of all colposcopes. Special rubber cups may be fitted to the eyepiece for eyeglass wearers to prevent damage to their lenses. The angle of the eyepieces relative to the long axis of the instrument is variable and should be tested individually for comfort and ease of viewing (*see* Figure 2–2).

Filters

Colposcopes are usually provided with a green (less often blue) filter that is interposed between the light source and the viewing area. The filter absorbs red from the color spectrum, thus permitting blood vessels to stand out in detail as black structures. Contrast between normal and abnormal epithelia is also enhanced with the use of the filter.

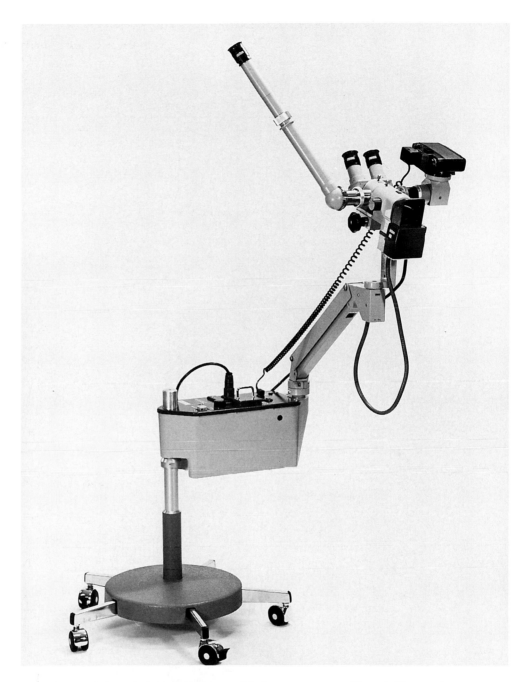

Figure 2-2. Zeiss photocolposcope with four-step magnifier. A fiberoptic cable and halogen lighting are part of the colposcope. A teaching tube and a camera are attached.

Light Source

The light source is frequently an incandescent bulb with a rheostat to alter the light intensity. The bulb strength may vary from 6 to 12 volts and 30 to 50 watts. A tungsten halogen lamp may be substituted for the incandescent bulb. The illumination of the tungsten halogen lamp may be adjusted by a potentiometer and brought to the instrument through a fiberoptic cable. Fiberoptic lighting tends to be cooler for both the patient and the colposcopist.

TABLE 2-1. OBJECTIVES, MAGNIFICATIONS, AND FIELD OF VIEW DIAMETERS

Objective Length (mm)	Focal Working Distance (cm)	12.5[a] Eyepiece and 125 mm Length of Tube			
		Minimum Magnification	Maximum Magnification	Maximum Field of View (mm)	Minimum Field of View (mm)
200	20	3.1	20	66	10
250	25	2.5	16	82	12.5
300	30	2.1	14	96	14.2
350	35	1.8	11.2	112	18
400	40	1.6	10	128	20

[a] 10× Eyepiece multiply magnification by 0.8. 16× Eyepiece multiply magnification by 1.28. 20× Eyepiece multiply magnification by 1.6.
Reproduced with permission from Carl Zeiss, West Germany.

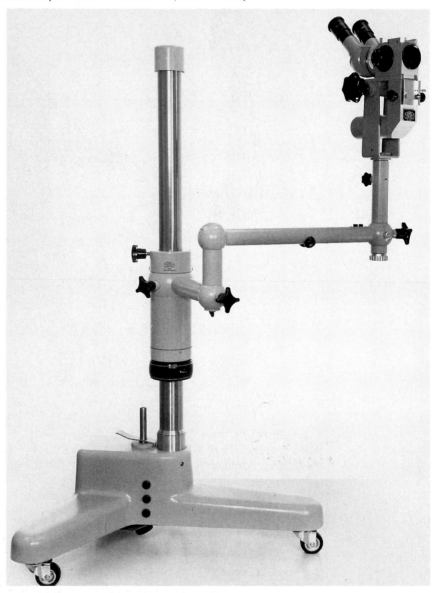

Figure 2-3. Zeiss colposcope 1 on heavy mobile base. The transformer for lighting is in the base.

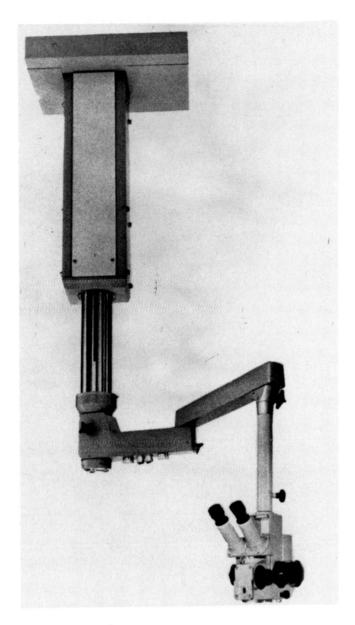

Figure 2-4. Zeiss colposcope 1 on a ceiling mount.

Stands

The colposcope may be placed on an adjustable stand with a transformer in the base (Figure 2-3), affixed to the side of an examining table, or attached to a wall or even the ceiling. Some ceiling mounts may have electrohydraulic capabilities for raising and lowering the scope (Figure 2-4). Attachment to the examining table seems preferable for a gynecologist's private office. If the colposcope is to be used in more than one room, a simple mobile stand may be purchased so that the colposcope can be transported readily from room to room (Figure 2-5).

The stands vary from the simple to the complex. The simple stands, which may have either a flat base or wheels, are easy to store; however, unless the wheels have a locking mechanism, they tend to be unstable and tend to make it difficult to keep the colposcope in focus (*see* Figure 2-3). It is imperative that the stands equipped with wheels have a wheel locking mechanism or be heavy enough so that once the colposcope is focused, it will remain so throughout the examination. Instruments with overhead

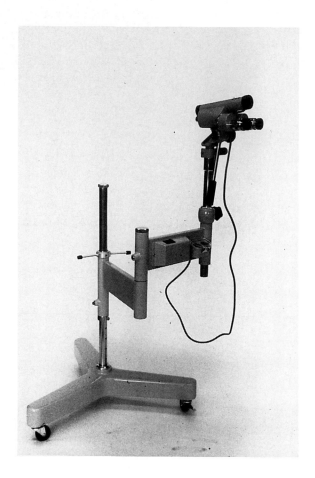

Figure 2-5. Fixed focus colposcope on a simple wheel base.

gantries may also have problems with stability, especially if they are used in conjunction with a laser apparatus.

Before purchasing a colposcope, the physician must determine the purposes for which the instrument will be used. If only the cervix is to be colposcoped, then a fairly simple instrument, with fixed focus magnification, will be sufficient. If the colposcope is to be used as an operating microscope for procedures involving the cervix, vagina, vulva, urethra, anus, and other mucous membranes, then multiple magnification is a necessity. If laser is part of the armamentarium of the gynecologist, then the instrument must have the capability of making use of special attachments to support this technique. In addition, if extensive teaching, video taping, and photographic record documentation of referred patients is necessary, the complexity of the instrument (and accordingly, the price) will be much greater (Figure 2–6).

COLPOSCOPIC TECHNIQUE

The Examination Table

Because the colposcopic examination is moderately time consuming, comfort is extremely important for both the patient, so that she cooperates during the examination, and the examiner, so that he or she does not develop neck or back difficulties at the end of a series of examinations. The ordinary gynecologic table is generally adequate to provide for the comfort of the patient. Special knee and calf supports are available that offer greater comfort than the ordinary heel support with which the usual table is equipped. Tables with automatic foot controls for height adjustment are almost a necessity in order to bring the patient's cervix, vagina, and vulva to the eye level of the examiner. The usual gynecologic table tends to be somewhat lower than is ideal, and the foot of the table may have to be raised with wooden blocks. Conversely, the examiner's stool must be capable of being lowered sufficiently to provide the proper sightline of the colposcopist with the lower genital tract.

Examination Materials

The materials necessary for the colposcopic examination should be on a stand beside the examiner. They include warm, various-sized and -shaped specula (such as the Graves and Pedersen), saline, 3% to 5% acetic acid, 50% Lugol's iodine, and large or small cotton-tipped swabs. In addition, either on the table or nearby, various instruments for performing biopsies (*see following section*) should be available (Figure 2–7).

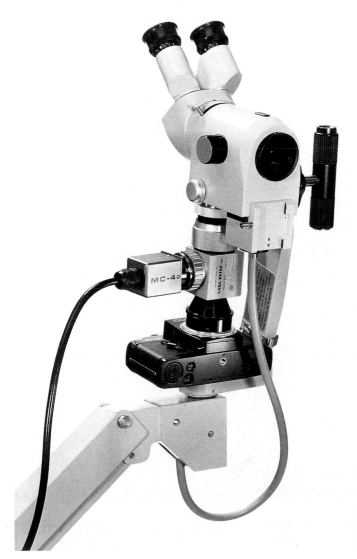

Figure 2–6. Zeiss colposcope with video camera and 35 mm camera attached.

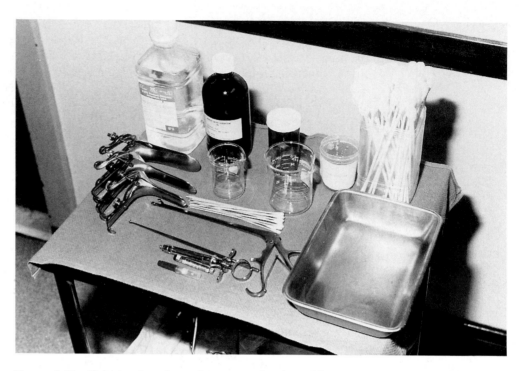

Figure 2-7. Table set-up for colposcopy. On the table are saline, acetic acid, Lugol's iodine, small and large cotton-tipped applicators, specula, hook, biopsy instruments, and local infiltration set.

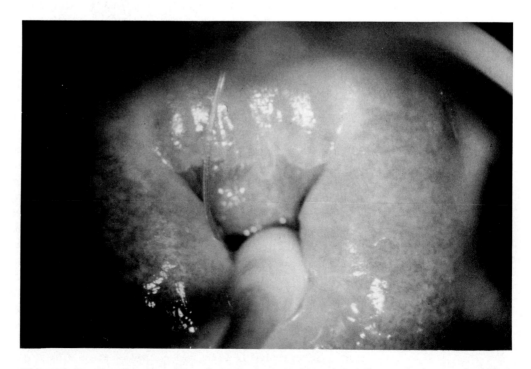

Figure 2-8. Small cotton-tipped applicator used to retract the posterior cervical lip to visualize the squamocolumnar junction and endocervical canal.

The Colposcopic Examination

The examination should proceed in an orderly fashion. After the speculum has been inserted, it is held by one hand and manipulated so that the cervix is at a right angle to the light of the colposcope. The other hand should then bring the colposcope toward the area of examination until it is in proper view. Next, mucus should be gently removed from the cervix with either a dry cotton-tipped applicator or one that has been soaked in normal saline. First the cervix, then the vagina and vulva are inspected using a 5× to 10× magnification initially. The cervical and vaginal surfaces should be moistened with normal saline in order to view their vascular patterns because a dry epithelial surface does not give a satisfactory view of these patterns. Gross lesions, vascular detail, and opacity of the epithelium can be ascertained at this initial examination. The green filter should then be interposed between the light and the viewing field so that the vascular changes will appear as black structures against a background of transluscent epithelium. Occasionally, abnormal epithelium also will stand out from the surrounding normal epithelium when the filter is in place.

A 3% to 5% solution of acetic acid is then gently applied to the surface being viewed, using soaked, cotton-tipped applicators. The best technique is to compress the soaked applicators so that the solution runs over the epithelial surface, rather than using a rubbing or patting motion, which may cause abrasion of the epithelium and interfere with proper evaluation of the surface. The 5% solution, if allowed to remain in contact with the mucous membrane, may elicit a complaint from the patient of a burning sensation. If the milder dilutions are used, however, one must keep in mind that abnormalities may take a few moments longer to develop than with the use of the 5% solution. The aceto-white changes in the epithelial surfaces are transient: they develop within one minute after application of the milder solutions and fade within two to three minutes. They can be restored with another application of the acetic acid. Several applications of the solution may be required during the course of a single examination.

Tissues treated with acetic acid should be inspected under 5 to 16 magnification. If abnormal vessels are seen, better contrast is achieved by using the green filter and by increasing magnification to 25× or even 40×. The portio of the cervix and the visible portion of the endocervical canal should be inspected in a systematic fashion circumferentially around the os of the cervix. A small cotton-tipped applicator soaked in the acetic acid may be utilized to examine the endocervical canal (Figure 2–8). An Iris hook may also be used, although it will often cause some bleeding that will interfere with adequate visualization (Figure 2–9). If the upper endocervical canal is to be examined, a variety of endocervical specula can be utilized. They are available in numerous shapes, sizes, and widths with a variety of ratchet mechanisms between the handles to keep the specula in place (Figure 2–10, Figure 2–11). With the aid of an endocervical speculum, at least 1.5 cm of the endocervical canal can be observed in most patients; in many parous individuals the entire endocervical canal can be seen (Figure 2–12).

Many colposcopists, especially those in Europe and South America, advise that iodine staining of the mucosa should be the final step in every colposcopic examination. The solutions usually used are Schiller's (1 gm pure iodine and 2 gms Kl in 300 mL water) and Lugol's (5% iodine and 10% Kl in water). The iodine solution must be aqueous, because an alcohol base causes destruction of the mucosal surface that hinders the pathologic evaluation of biopsies. Lugol's iodine solution is often used in a 50% dilution rather than full strength. Native, mature squamous epithelium high in glycogen content stains deep mahogany brown when iodine is applied to it, a finding referred to as a Schiller negative or iodine positive area. Columnar epithelium, atrophic squamous epithelium, undifferentiated metaplastic epithelium, and dysplastic epithelium, in general, are nonglycogenated and, therefore, do not stain with iodine (Figure 2–13).

Many expert colposcopists feel that the iodine test on the cervix adds little or nothing to the evaluation of the colposcopic picture. It destroys the minute details so useful in

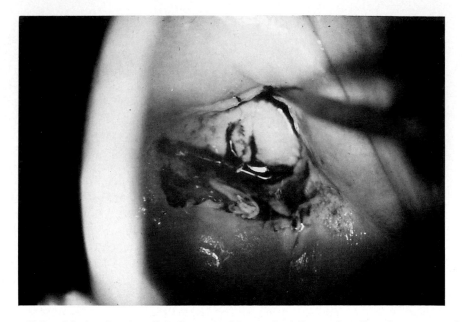

Figure 2-9. Iris hook retracting the anterior cervical lip to visualize the extent of the lesion.

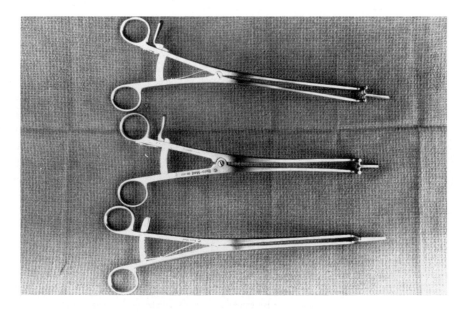

Figure 2-10. Endocervical specula.

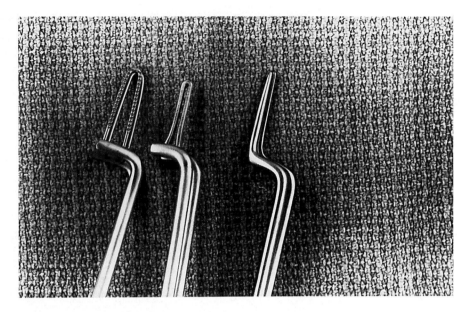

Figure 2-11. Tips of endocervical specula, from left to right, for parous, nulliparous, and stenotic cervices.

localizing the most abnormal areas for directed biopsies. Also, because of the nonspecificity of the test, both malignant and benign areas may produce a positive result. Interest, however, in the iodine-staining methodology as a technique to distinguish the ordinary human papilloma virus (HPV) lesions from more significant dysplastic lesions has caused a renewed interest in the use of the iodine-staining technique (*see* Chapter 10). In the colposcopic examination of the vagina the use of iodine staining is of inestimable value.

BIOPSY TECHNIQUES

The goal of the colposcopic examination is to determine the area or areas of greatest possible abnormality. To verify the clinical impression, tissue sampling of specific abnormal areas must be done under colposcopic guidance. The colposcopist should observe through the colposcope and watch the head of the biopsy instrument as he or she takes the samples of tissue. If for any reason the examiner cannot do this, the area to be biopsied should be marked with the end of a cotton-tipped applicator dipped in Lugol's iodine solution (Figure 2-14). After taking the biopsy specimens, the examiner should visualize the sampled area with the colposcope to be certain that the biopsy instrument indeed removed the marked areas (Figure 2-15). Frequent biopsying during the early part of training in colposcopy is necessary to achieve a clear understanding of the underlying histopathology. Multiple biopsies, properly labeled (*described later*), allow the colposcopist to hone his or her expertise in correlating specific colposcopic images with histologic patterns.

Biopsy Forceps

Carefully excised, well-oriented, and properly fixed specimens permit the most accurate diagnoses. The common instruments for removing small bites of tissue include the Ep-

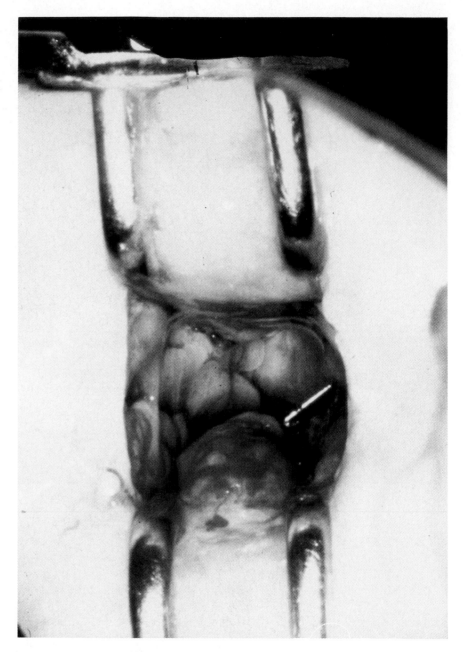

Figure 2-12.   Colpophotograph of the endocervix being viewed through an endocervical speculum. The canal is visualized for at least 1.5 cm. Note the broad endocervical folds.

pendorfer, Kevorkian, Young, Tischler, and Burke biopsy forceps (Figure 2–16, Figure 2–17). The Eppendorfer, Kevorkian, and Young instruments take small, relatively superficial, samples. Unless the examiner stablizes the cervix, they tend to slip off and the resulting sample is unsatisfactory (Figure 2–18). These instruments, not infrequently, crush rather than cut through the epithelium, producing an unsatisfactory specimen (Figure 2–19). They may be expeditiously used on the pregnant cervix or for vaginal and vulvar sampling.

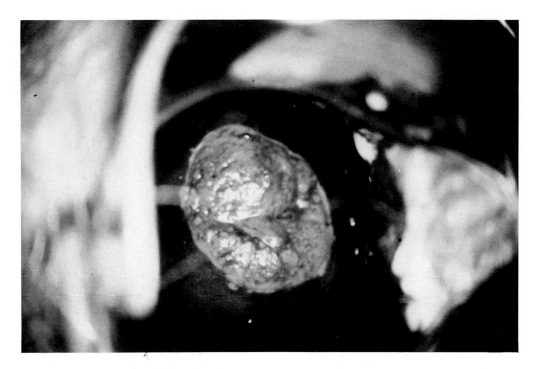

Figure 2-13. Cervix after staining with 50% Lugol's iodine solution. The stratified squamous epithelium stains intensely; the columnar epithelium does not take the stain.

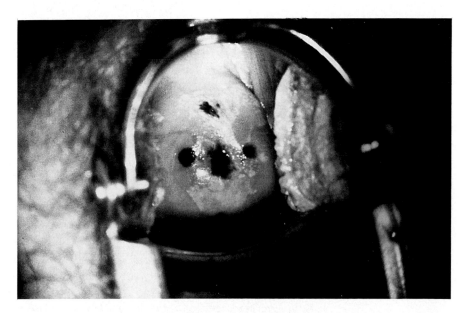

Figure 2-14. Colpophotograph of a cervical lesion being marked before biopsy with Lugol's iodine.

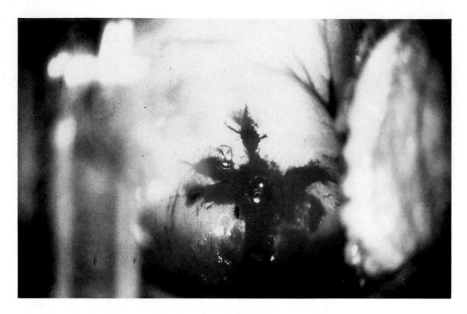

Figure 2–15.   Cervix in Figure 2–14 after biopsy. The biopsies have sampled the marked fields.

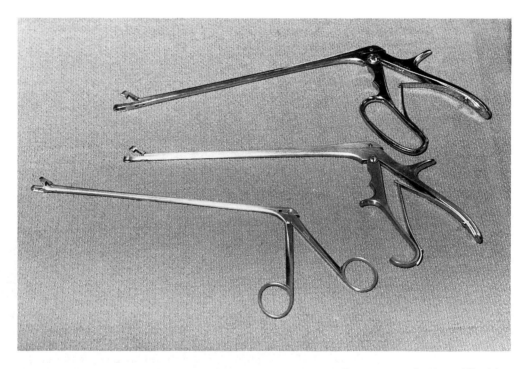

Figure 2–16.   Biopsy forceps used during colposcopy. From top to bottom: Tischler, Burke, and Eppendorfer biopsy forceps.

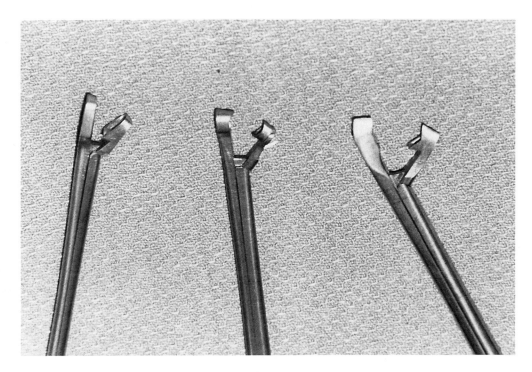

Figure 2-17. View of biopsy forceps, left to right: Eppendorfer, Burke, and Tischler biopsy forceps.

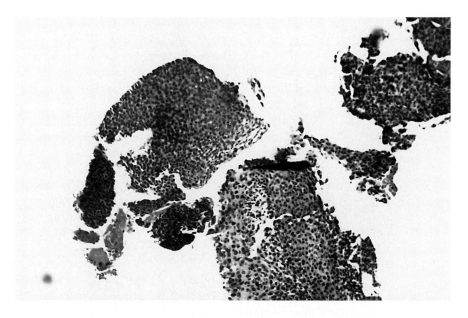

Figure 2-18. Unsatisfactory cervical biopsy specimen. The biopsy contains cervical intraepithelial neoplasia, but the fragments are small, poorly oriented, and contain no stroma. Therefore cervical intraepithelial neoplasia cannot be graded and invasion cannot be evaluated.

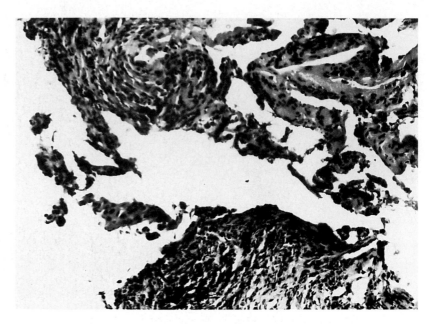

Figure 2–19. Cervical biopsy specimen with crushed artifact. Both the epithelium *(upper)* and stroma *(bottom)* are so distorted that evaluation is not possible.

The Kevorkian and Young forceps have serrations on the posterior blade that aid in stablizing the area requiring biopsy. The Tischler and Burke biopsy forceps have a projection on each blade that acts as a stabilizing tooth so that additional immobilization of the cervix is hardly ever necessary (*see* Figure 2–17). The Tischler head is 5 × 5 × 4 mm. This instrument does take a nice longitudinal sample; however, there is a tendency to take too deep a biopsy with resultant excessive bleeding. The Burke biopsy forceps, whose head measures 5 × 4 × 3 mm, was designed to obviate the problem of depth. It takes a biopsy that extends only 2 mm in depth, but this is adequate to obtain tissue from not only the epithelium but also the underlying stroma (Figure 2–20, Figure 2–21). Care should be taken that the cutting edges of the biopsy forceps are not dulled by misuse. Forceps should not be autoclaved; they should be soaked in Cidex or sterilized with gas. If they become dulled, they may either be sent back to the manufacturer for resharpening or the clinician may sharpen them, using a jeweler's file, with the colposcope as a magnifier.

Obtaining biopsy specimens may be facilitated by stabilizing the cervix or vagina by using a fine hook such as the Iris or Burke hooks (Figure 2–22). The hook holds the cervix firmly or tents the epithelium of the vagina so that the biopsy forceps can be applied perpendicular to the fold and an adequate specimen taken. A preferable method of vaginal biopsy is to inject a small wheal of saline underneath the epithelium, thus tenting it so that the top of the wheal can be removed readily with the biopsy forceps. This technique, however, will limit somewhat the amount of underlying connective tissue that is removed from the vagina.

Obtaining and Labeling Specimens

The biopsy should be taken to a depth sufficient to obtain enough stroma for differential diagnosis (Figure 2–23). The epithelium must be cut at right angles to the surface in order to avoid tangential sections. Biopsies can be submitted to the pathologist floating free in separately labeled jars of formalin. They should never all be placed in one jar, since the colposcopist would then have no way of correlating his or her clinical impression of the area from which the biopsy was taken with the pathology report. The various specimen jars should be labeled by the numbers of the clock or by describ-

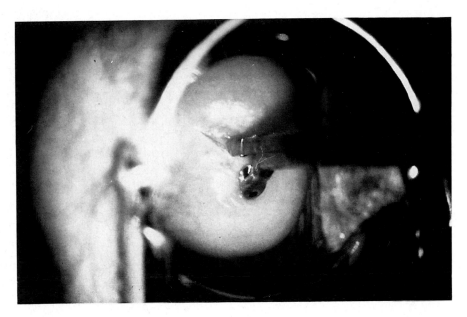

Figure 2-20. Burke biopsy forceps sampling the anterior lip of the cervix.

ing the area of the cervix, vagina, or vulva from which the biopsy was taken. In order to conserve jars, several specimens may be placed within the same container if each specimen is individually wrapped and labeled. A technique utilized by the senior author involves placing the specimen between two pieces of thin styrofoam, which are then held together with paper clips or staples (Figure 2–24, Figure 2–25). The styrofoam circles must be labeled with water-insoluble ink, which will not wash off when the circles are placed in fixative. A Sharpie pen satisfies this requirement of water insolubility. Specimens must never be placed in saline as the surface epithelium may be destroyed, thus obviating adequate histologic diagnosis.

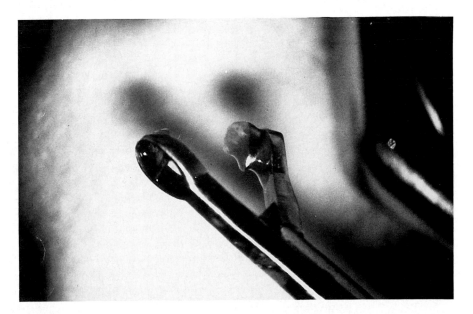

Figure 2-21. Biopsy of Figure 2-20. The specimen can be seen in the anterior jaw of the forceps.

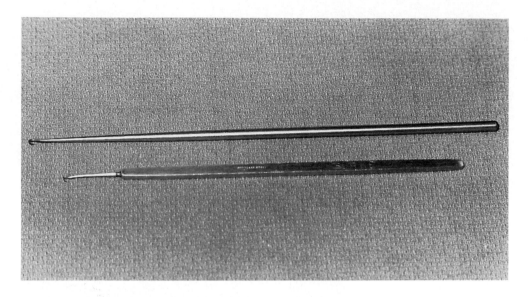

Figure 2-22. Hooks used to manipulate tissue. Top to bottom: Burke and Iris.

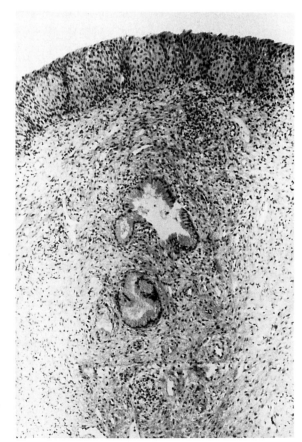

Figure 2-23. Well-oriented biopsy specimen with adequate stroma.

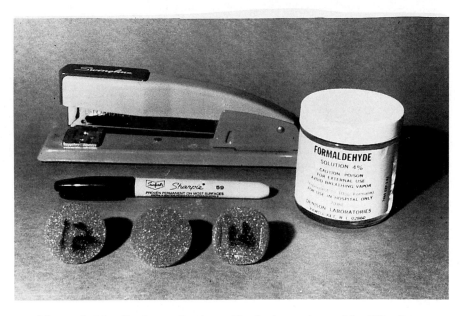

Figure 2-24. Senior author's method of specimen identification.

Hemostasis

Hemostasis is obtained by applying Monsel's solution (ferric subsulfate) followed by a gentle pressure of the cotton-tipped applicator. The Monsel's solution should be allowed to remain in a wide necked jar until its consistency is that of mustard, at which time its efficiency as a hemostatic will be markedly improved. Silver nitrate, either on sticks or in solution, may also be used for hemostasis; however, it has the disadvantage of leaving small deposits of silver that may interfere with subsequent colposcopic evaluation of the area. Although some colposcopists have used the nasal-tip cautery at the base of the biopsy site for hemostasis, we believe it is relatively contraindicated. Cautery destroys the surrounding tissue and renders it unsuitable for later histologic or colposcopic examination.

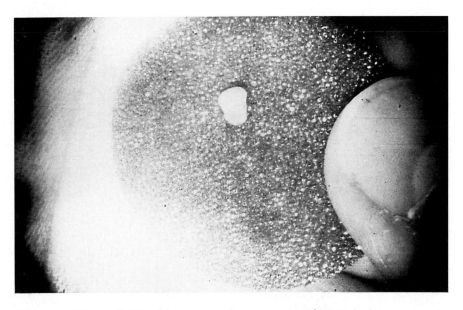

Figure 2-25. Biopsy specimen on styrofoam circles.

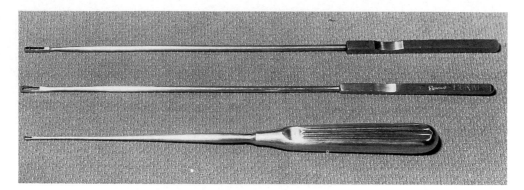

Figure 2-26. Endocervical curettes.

ENDOCERVICAL CURETTAGE

As part of the colposcopic technique, endocervical curettage (ECC) may have to be performed. Endocervical curettage is a procedure that evokes a moderate amount of discussion by colposcopists. Endocervical curettage is indicated if a lesion extends up the canal, if its upper edge cannot be biopsied, or if the colposcopic examination is unsatisfactory (squamocolumnar junction cannot be seen in its entirety). The routine use of ECC, however, following a satisfactory colposcopic examination may sometimes produce false-positive results resulting in needless excisional conization. Those workers who advocate the routine use of ECC following the colposcopic examination feel that, in marginal cases, invasive squamous cell carcinoma may be detected with this procedure. The use of ECC will be discussed in greater detail in Chapter 13.

To perform the ECC, the usual instrument is either the Kevorkian endocervical curette or, more recently, one of several smaller endocervical curettes (Figure 2-26, Figure 2-27). The latter have been devised to prevent sampling of the lesion on the portio as the curette is brought down from the canal. In general, when the ECC is done, the canal

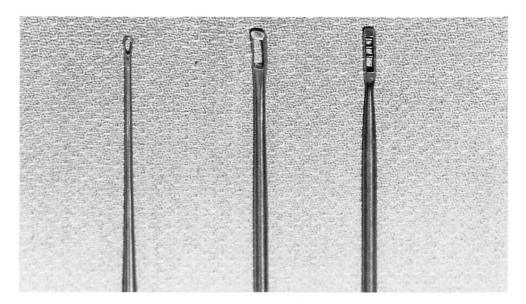

Figure 2-27.   View of heads of endocervical curettes, demonstrating variation in sizes and presence or absence of baskets.

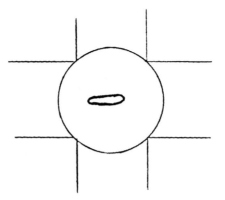

Figure 2-28.   Simple drawing used by senior author to document colposcopic findings.

should be sampled without withdrawing the curette to minimize the possibility of contaminating the sample with a strip of abnormal epithelium from the portio of the cervix. The specimen should be collected on either pieces of filter paper or telfa gauze and placed in formalin. All of the blood and mucus as well as the fragments of tissue should be removed with fine nasal bayonet forceps to be sure that an adequate amount of tissue is obtained. In performing the curettage, one should aim to obtain not only the surface epithelium but the underlying stroma as well in order to make the evaluation meaningful.

RECORDING DATA

Precise recording of data is essential to good colposcopic technique. Obviously, photography at the time of colposcopy is the most accurate method of recording the findings. There are, however, several graphic methods, which when accompanied by a written descriptive narrative of the findings, are adequate to record the data. The simplest is one in which a circle representing the portio and endocervical canal is utilized, with four-quadrant extensions representing the vagina (Figure 2–28). Arrows localizing the findings, with descriptions amplified in the narrative, are used. A more complex type of diagram in which the cervix is divided into concentric circles in multiple sections is available (Figure 2–29). Other sophisticated systems have been devised, but the senior author finds them cumbersome and no better than the simplest methodology just described. A rudimentary hand drawing of the cervix and vagina, with a clear explanation of the findings and a list of biopsy sites, is sufficient for most record keeping.

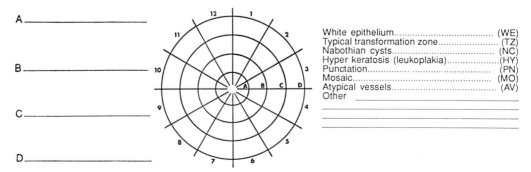

Figure 2-29.   Alternate method of documenting colposcopic findings using preprinted diagrams.

Chapter 3 | The Normal Cervix

In the newborn female the vagina and cervix are covered by two epithelia called the *original* (or *native*) *stratified squamous epithelium* and the *original* (or *native*) *columnar epithelium*. Normally the stratified squamous epithelium covers the vagina and most of the cervix whereas the columnar epithelium covers the surface of the endocervical canal (Figure 3–1). In the fetus the vagina and cervix are derived from the fused distal ends of the mullerian ducts and are lined by a single layer of mullerian-type columnar epithelium. During the first half of intrauterine development, this columnar epithelium is replaced by the upward growth of stratified squamous epithelium originating in the urogenital sinus to a point usually at or near the external cervical os (Figure 3–2). The original or native columnar epithelium lines the endocervical canal, and sometimes the inner part of the cervical portio; it is contiguous with the endometrium at the internal cervical os.

HISTOLOGY AND CYTOLOGY OF THE EXOCERVICAL MUCOSA

The stratified squamous epithelium of the cervix presents a characteristic appearance of increasing maturation from the basal layer to the surface, accompanied by cytoplasmic glycogen accumulation, which is the basis for the staining of the epithelium when it is exposed to Schiller's or Lugol's iodine solution (*see* Figure 2–13). The multilayered squamous epithelium of the exocervix originates from the basal layer, which rests on a thin basement lamina. Normally only one or two layers thick, the basal zone is mitotically active and formed of small cuboidal cells with round central nuclei; ultrastructurally, cytoplasmic organelles are sparse and intercellular bridges (desmosomes) are relatively infrequent. During upward growth and maturation, the cells change significantly: the cell nuclei become pyknotic; the cytoplasm increases in volume and becomes pale, staining secondary to the accumulation of glycogen; and the orientation of the cells changes from a vertical to a horizontal axis. The nuclear:cytoplasmic ratio markedly decreases, and the cell shape also changes from round to elliptic, so that the upper layers of the epithelium have a "basket weave" appearance (Figure 3–3). Based on the size and shape of the cell, the size of the nucleus, and the amount and density of the cytoplasm, the maturing cells have been classified in order of increasing maturation as parabasal, intermediate, and superficial (Figure 3–4).

The full spectrum of squamous maturation is dependent on the presence of estrogen. During the relative estrogen deficiencies, before puberty and after the menopause, the epithelium consists predominantly of basal and parabasal cells.

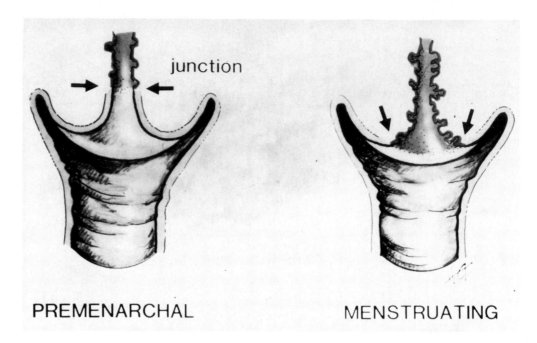

junction

PREMENARCHAL   MENSTRUATING

Figure 3-1. Diagram showing the location of the squamocolumnar junction at the anatomic external os of the cervix prior to menarche and the location on the portio during the menstrual life of women *(arrow)*.

At the ultrastructural level maturation and senescence are characterized by collapse of nuclear chromatin, with a decrease in nuclear size, and by accumulation of finely granular glycogen particles in the cytoplasm. In addition, there are increases in cytoplasmic filaments of the keratin protein type, increased intercellular desmosomes, and formation of a submembraneous and intracytoplasmic cytoskeleton that confers structural rigidity to the cell. When the original squamous epithelium is subjected to scanning electron microscopy, a characteristic appearance is seen (Figure 3–5). The superficial cells are flat and polygonal with a central raised area representing the nucleus. The cell borders are distinct and raised. At higher magnification, numerous microridges are often seen beneath the surface membrane (Figure 3–6); these microridges may represent the internal cytoskeleton.

Cytologic smears contain a sampling of those cells forming the uppermost layers of the cervix and thus reflect the most mature elements in the epithelium. During active reproductive life, the superficial and intermediate squamous cells are the most common types noted in scrapings from the exocervix or vagina. Superficial cells are large, polygonal, and thin, with well-defined cytoplasmic borders. Nuclei are pyknotic, variably dense, and centrally located. Due to its thinness, the cytoplasm is virtually transparent, being pink or green-blue with the stains typically used to prepare smears (Figure 3–7).

Intermediate cells are also polygonal, but compared to the superficial cells they are smaller, have larger nuclei with finely dispersed chromatin and a female sex chromatin mass, are more dense, and have deeply stained blue or red cytoplasm (Figure 3–8). Basal and parabasal cells are the most prevalent or only elements in the smear of atrophic cervical and vaginal mucosa (as typically present in premenarchal and postmenopausal women). They are small, round to oval cells having large, relatively open nuclei with

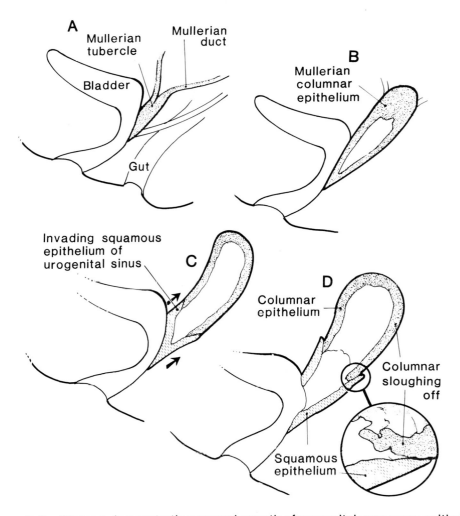

Figure 3-2. Diagram demonstrating upward growth of urogenital squamous epithelium during the first half of intrauterine development.

a diffuse chromatin pattern and very dense green-blue cytoplasm (Figure 3–9). Occasionally, the postmenopausal atrophic smear will contain cells pleomorphic in size, shape, and nuclear pattern with cytoplasmic staining suggestive of keratinization. Such cells can mimic those of squamous neoplasia, but their true nature can be elucidated by their disappearance after a trial of topical estrogen cream used on the cervicovaginal mucosa (Figure 3–10).

HISTOLOGY AND CYTOLOGY OF THE ENDOCERVICAL MUCOSA

The normal endocervical epithelium is a single layer of tall columnar cells lining the surface of the endocervical canal (Figure 3–11). This epithelium is arranged into numerous folds and crypts as described by Fluhmann (Figure 3–12). Smaller folds are formed from many large folds, a feature especially prominent adjacent to the external os of the cervical canal. When reviewed in cross section in histologic specimens, they have the appearance of a gland, and thus, the term "endocervical glands" is erroneously applied to these crypts (Figure 3–13). The majority of the cells lining the surface have basal nuclei and pale apical cytoplasm containing mucin; ultrastructurally, the cells are characterized by surface microvilli and by features typical of active secretory cells: prominent,

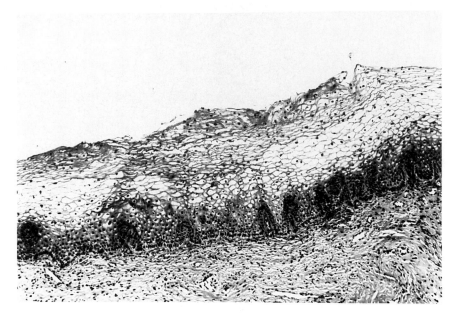

Figure 3–3. Histology of normal stratified squamous epithelium of the exocervix. The squamous mucosa shows orderly maturation from small basal cells that lie adjacent to the stroma, to cells with copious cytoplasm and small nuclei at the surface. Note the characteristic "basket weave" appearance of the interdigitating maturing cells. The stroma extends into the epithelium as short papillae at the base of the mucosa.

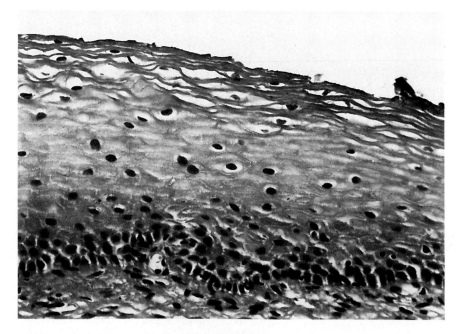

Figure 3–4. High power photomicrograph of squamous mucosa. At the base, there are two rows of basal cells characterized by small, round nuclei and a high nuclear: cytoplasmic ratio. Above the basal zone, the cells mature, acquiring cytoplasmic glycogen and demonstrating nuclear pyknosis. At the surface, the superficial cells have inconspicuous nuclei in a horizontal orientation.

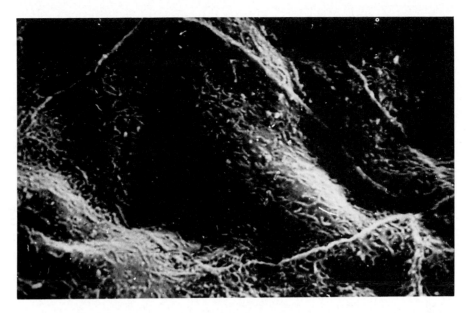

Figure 3-5. Scanning electron micrograph of surface of superficial squamous cells of exocervix. The lateral cell border is delineated by a distinct ridge. The cell surface contains microridges. *(Courtesy of Joseph Jordan.)*

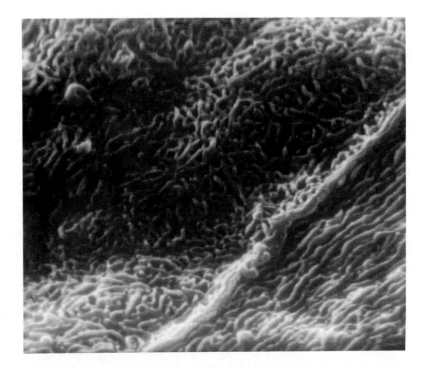

Figure 3-6. Higher magnification of scanning electron micrograph of Figure 3-5 showing surface microridges. *(Reprinted with permission from* The Cervix, *by J Jordan and A Singer.)*

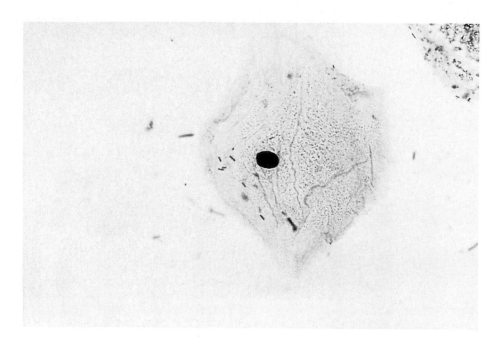

Figure 3-7.   Cytology of a normal squamous superficial cell.

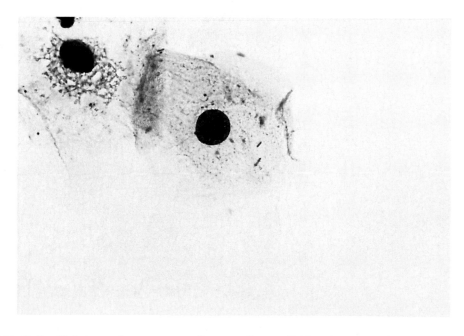

Figure 3-8.   Cytology of a squamous intermediate cell. Note larger nucleus with a more open chromatin appearance and increased nuclear:cytoplasmic ratio.

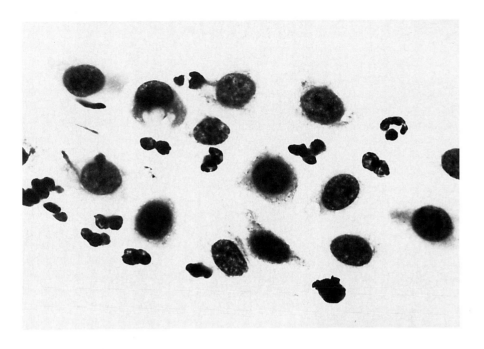

Figure 3-9. Cytosmear with basal and parabasal cells.

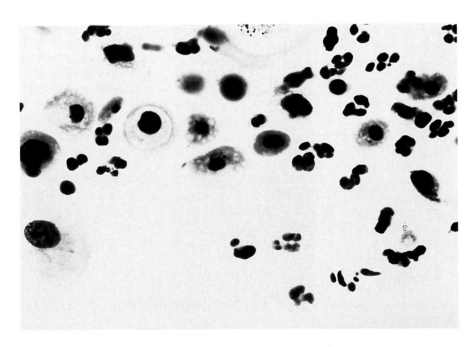

Figure 3-10. Cytologic appearance of atrophy. The parabasal cells bear a resemblance to the cells seen in atypical parakeratosis.

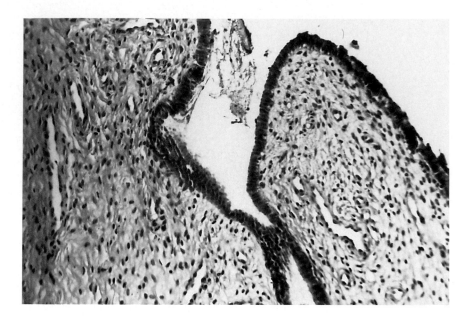

Figure 3-11. Sagittal section of normal endocervix. The surface is lined by a single row of columnar cells that extend into the stroma in the form of invaginations.

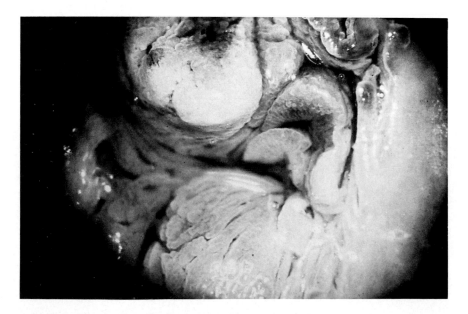

Figure 3-12. Colpophotograph of endocervical folds. Note the pattern of arborization on the posterior lip of the cervix as the folds approach the surface. *(Reprinted with permission from* Basic and Advanced Laser Surgery in Gynecology, *by MS Baggish.)*

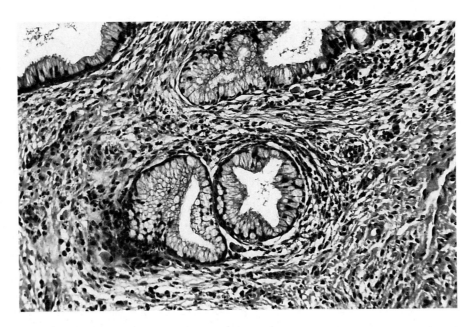

Figure 3-13. Cross section of normal endocervix. In this plane of the section the endocervical invaginations appear as "glands."

subnuclear, rough endoplasmic reticulum, a supranuclear Golgi zone, and numerous, apical, membrane-bound secretory vacuoles. A minority of the columnar cells are nonsecretory and have long surface cilia; cells of this type are found throughout the mullerian duct system, most prominently in the fallopian tubes (Figure 3-14).

In cytologic smears, the columnar cells may be present singly, in strips, or in sheets. When viewed parallel to their long axis, the cells form a row with a "picket fence" appearance (Figure 3-15). In cross section, each cell has a polygonal shape; in sheets, the cells form a honeycomb or mosaic configuration (Figure 3-16). Most of the cells will be mucinous, with vacuolated or granular, pale apical cytoplasm; the remaining cells will have apical cilia and more homogenous cytoplasm. In both types of columnar cells, the nuclei are basal, round or oval, and have finely dispersed chromatin. Multiple small nucleoli are usually present as well.

The original columnar epithelium demonstrated its characteristic appearance when viewed by scanning electron microscopy (Figure 3-17). Fingerlike villi with deep clefts are present. Each villus is covered by polygonal cells that are about 4 μ in diameter. The cells tend to be uniform in size and closely packed. Ciliated cells may be seen interspersed among the mucus secreting cells.

SQUAMOCOLUMNAR JUNCTION

The interface of these two original epithelia is called the *squamocolumnar junction,* (Figure 3-18a, Figure 3-18b). Although it is described as being located at the external os of the cervix, examination of the cervices of women at different ages shows that the area of the squamocolumnar junction moves in relationship to the presence or absence of estrogen (Figure 3-19). Neonates will have the squamocolumnar junction closer to the portio of the cervix than to the canal due to the influence of intrauterine maternal estrogen. In the premenarchal stage, the squamocolumnar junction is more likely to appear at the anatomical external os. At menarche and first pregnancy, both characterized by high serum estrogen levels, the squamocolumnar junction is on the cervical portio, where it remains throughout the woman's menstruating lifetime. It recedes up the canal in the postmenopausal state.

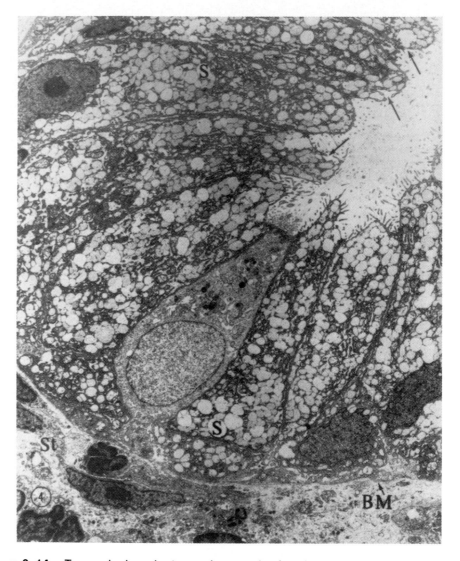

Figure 3-14. Transmission electron micrograph of endocervical epithelium. Most of the cells are mucinous type, with apical vacuoles. In the center is a ciliated cell. *(Reprinted with permission from* The Cervix *by J Jordan and A Singer.)*

As noted above, the various locations of the squamocolumnar junction are secondary to effects of estrogen, which causes a rearrangement and increased mass of mesenchymal elements within the cervical stroma. This remodeling results in an eversion of the cervix so that the columnar epithelium is brought into contact with the environment of the vagina. With the withdrawal of the estrogenic hormonal stimulus, the cervical stroma involutes and the columnar epithelium and squamocolumnar junction recede into the endocervical canal.

COLPOSCOPY OF THE NORMAL CERVIX

Two factors determine the colpscopic appearance of the original stratified squamous epithelium (*see* Chapter 1):

1. The cellular arrangement of the epithelium.
2. The nature of the underlying stroma.

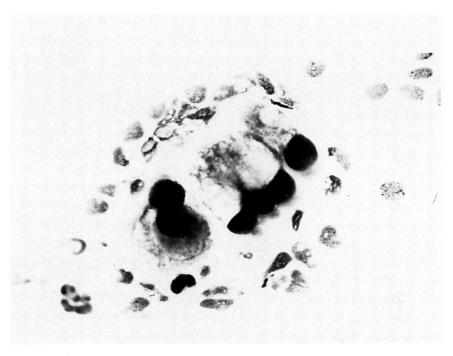

Figure 3-15. Endocervical cells in a palisade or picket fence arrangement as seen in cytosmears.

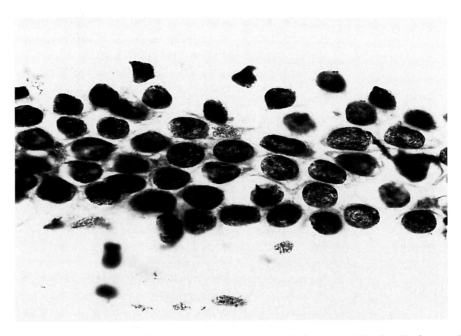

Figure 3-16. The mosaic or honeycomb arrangement of endocervical cells from a Pap smear.

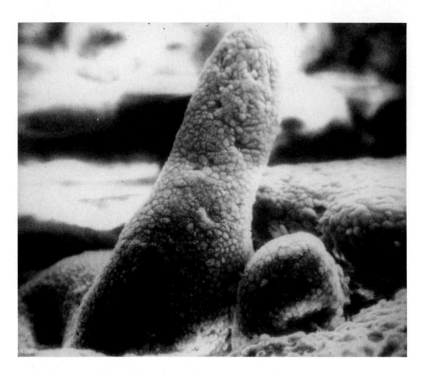

Figure 3-17.   Scanning electron micrograph of endocervical villus covered by columnar cells. *(Courtesy of Joseph Jordan.)*

The original stratified squamous epithelium is pink, translucent, flat, and relatively smooth (Figure 3-20). Its colposcopic characteristics are defined by the vessels in the lamina propria since the epithelium itself has no blood vessels.

Zinzer and Rosenbauer injected white latex into the vascular tree of the cervix and showed that there were four zones of terminal vessels in the lamina propria (Figure 3-21). The first and deepest zone, located at approximately 5 mm in depth, is a plexus of relatively large, freely anastomosing vessels. These continue upwards into a second zone of palisadelike vessels coursing perpendicularly or obliquely to the surface. The palisading vessels branch into the third zone of small vessels, called the basal network, that run parallel to the surface. From the basal network emerges a fourth zone of terminal capillaries that surround the epithelial basement lamina. Depending on the thickness of the surface epithelium, the basal network and the subepithelial capillaries can be observed and studied using a magnification of 12.5 to 16.

The prominence of the vascular network will vary according to the different hormonal states that influence epithelial thickness and vessel number. The thicker the epithelium, the less likely that the vessel will be seen, whereas in atrophic epithelium the vessels will be more prominent. In the postmenopausal state the appearance of the epithelium is usually paler than normal due to a decrease in stromal vascularity. The few vessels present, however, will be very prominent. In addition, spiderlike vessels representing even deeper vascular channels can sometimes be seen beneath the network capillaries in very thin atrophic squamous epithelium.

When the connective tissue papillae of the squamous epithelium of the cervix and the vagina are poorly developed or absent, the stromal vasculature is flattened. Consequently, a meshwork or network of delicate capillaries is seen in which the vessels are usually 50 to 250 μ apart (Figure 3-22). If the stromal papillae are well developed, hairpin capillaries, formed by the ascending and descending branches of a capillary loop within a papilla, are observed. The extent of stromal papillation and the angle of observation determines whether or not such hairpin structures are seen in their entirety. Within

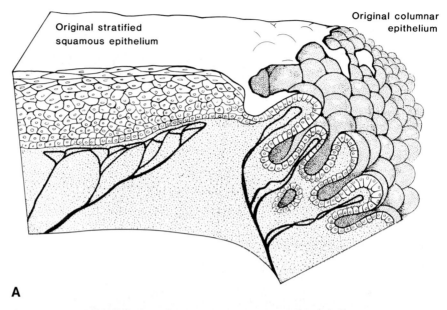

Original stratified
squamous epithelium

Original columnar
epithelium

A

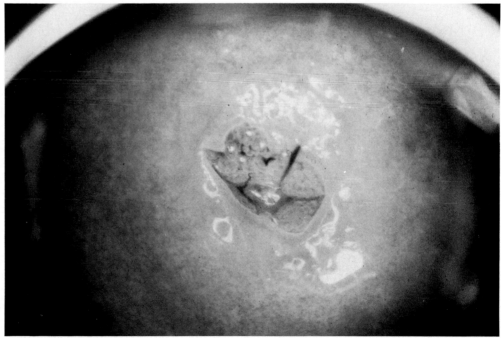

B

Figure 3-18.   A. Diagram of the anatomical squamocolumnar junction. **B.** Colpophotograph of the anatomical squamocolumnar junction. The original stratified squamous epithelium interfaces with the original columnar epithelium.

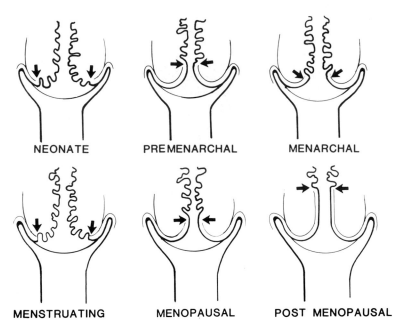

Figure 3–19. Diagram showing the location of the squamocolumnar junction during the lifetime of a woman.

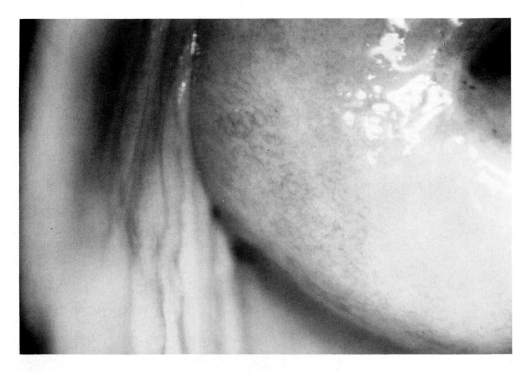

Figure 3–20. Colpophotograph of the original stratified squamous epithelium on the posterior lip of the cervix. The epithelium is smooth, flat, and some terminal vessels are present.

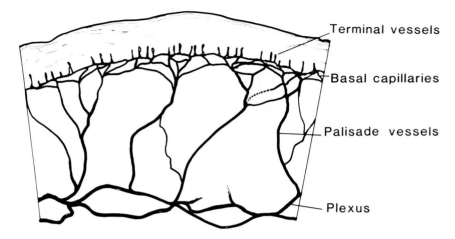

Figure 3-21. Diagramatic representation of the vascular arrangement of the native cervical squamous mucosa.

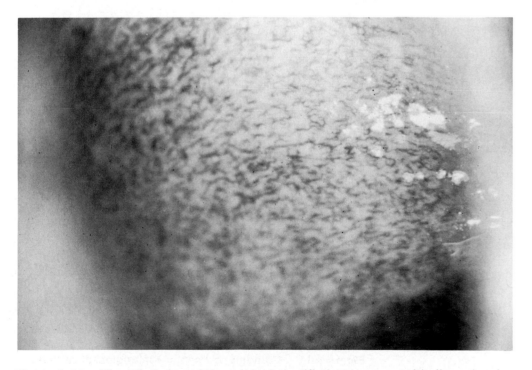

Figure 3-22. Magnified view of the original stratified squamous epithelium showing the terminal and network arborizing capillaries.

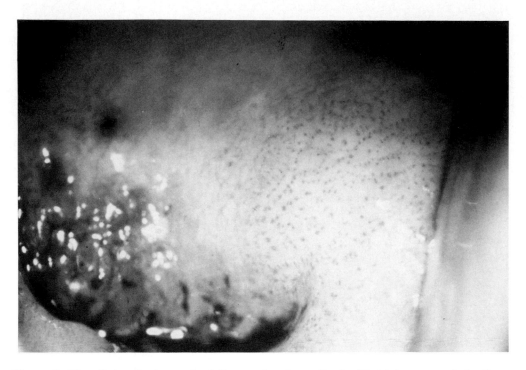

Figure 3-23. Colpophotograph of the cervix of a patient with trichomonas infection. Note presence of punctate vessels.

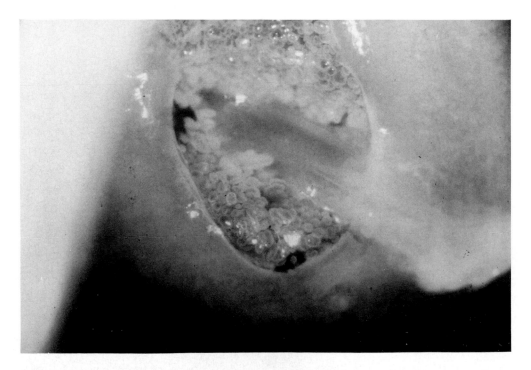

Figure 3-24. Colpophotograph of endocervix after application of acetic acid. Endocervical papillae adjacent to the exocervix have become swollen and grapelike. Note the mucus extruding from the os. *(Reprinted with permission from* Basic and Advanced Laser Surgery in Gynecology, *by MS Baggish.)*

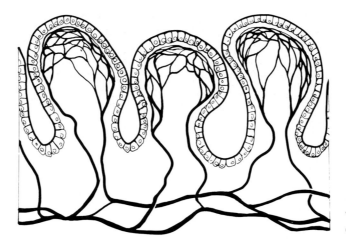

Figure 3-25. Diagram of the vascular network within the endocervical villi.

the same colposcopic section, hairpin vessels can be viewed tangentially as crests of loops or directly on end as fine punctate vessels; the latter will be noted especially during pregnancy and trichomonas infection (Figure 3–23, Color Plate 3).

Colposcopically the endocervix appears deep pink or red after cleansing with saline because of the single-layer nature of its columnar epithelium (Color Plate 4). This appearance is the result of the strong light of the colposcope traversing the epithelium and impinging on the vasculature present in the lamina propria. The folds or papillae of the columnar epithelium have a characteristic appearance when subjected to the usual colposcopic examination with acetic acid. Due to osmolar changes, the papillae adjacent to the exocervix swell and assume a characteristic grapelike appearance. The folds, however, tend to be broader and less grapelike in appearance within the endocervix itself (Figures 3–24, 3–25, 3–26).

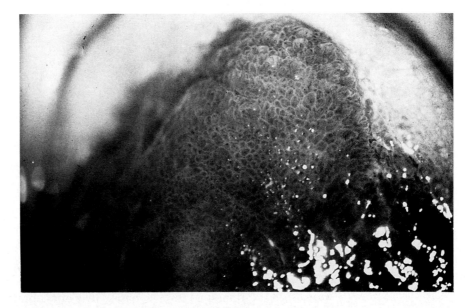

Figure 3-26. Colpophotograph of the anterior lip of the cervix, prior to the application of acetic acid, in diethylstilbestrol exposed woman. Note the dark vascular area within each villus.

The vascular network of the columnar epithelium is very complex. There are ascending and descending capillaries that intertwine at the top of the papillae forming a multi-channelled network (*see* Figure 3–25). These terminal capillary loops in each papilla are easily seen colposcopically (*see* Figure 3–26).

Chapter 4 | Normal Transformation Zone

THE SQUAMOCOLUMNAR JUNCTION

As noted in Chapter 3, at menarche the original squamocolumnar junction is normally transferred onto the cervical portio from its prepubertal location at or slightly inside the external os (*see* Figure 3–20). The movement of the squamocolumnar junction results from an estrogen-mediated increase in the volume of cervical stroma resulting in exposure of the endocervical columnar epithelium to the acid environment of the vagina. The original columnar epithelium is replaced by metaplastic squamous epithelium. The area of native columnar epithelium undergoing physiologic squamous metaplasia is termed the *transformation zone* (TZ) (Figure 4–1). The original squamocolumnar junction is therefore converted into a squamo-squamo junction composed of original and metaplastic squamous tissue. A new, more proximal, squamocolumnar junction develops between the original columnar epithelium and the transformed areas. This interface is called the physiologic squamocolumnar junction (Figure 4–2). This junction subsequently may be subject to a similar transformation process. The major significance of the TZ is that this area is the site of origin for virtually all cervical squamous dysplastic, in situ, and invasive lesions.

The normal physiologic transition from columnar to squamous epithelium is most active during three phases of life:

1. Intrauterine development and the neonatal period.
2. Menarche.
3. First pregnancy.

These periods represent times at which there are especially high levels of estrogen. Active metaplasia in the fetus takes place late in pregnancy (from 28 weeks to term) and has been attributed to the influence of the maternal steroids. With the withdrawal of maternal steroids after birth, the metaplastic process ceases. With the surge of estrogen that occurs at menarche and during the first pregnancy, the process is reactivated.

TOPOGRAPHY OF SQUAMOUS METAPLASIA IN THE TRANSFORMATION ZONE

Squamous metaplasia in the TZ is an irreversible process that tends to begin on, and be most prominent in, the tips and sides of the endocervical villi (Figure 4–3). The deeper parts of the villi and the endocervical clefts or invaginations are more variably involved. Residual clefts without metaplasia can be identified as gland openings in areas other-

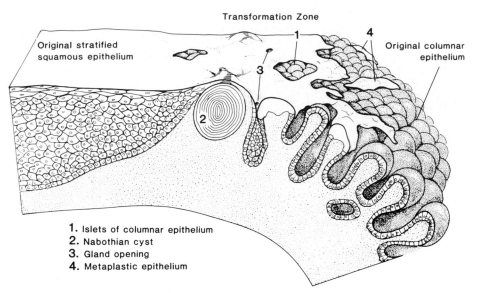

Figure 4-1. Diagram showing the transformation zone and the physiologic squamocolumnar junction.

wise showing squamous metaplasia (Figure 4–4). Nabothian cysts develop when the superficial portion of the endocervical cleft becomes occluded by the squamous metaplastic tissue, while columnar epithelium deep in the cleft continues to produce mucus (Figure 4–5).

In general, squamous metaplasia progresses from distal to more proximal zones within the TZ, but it does not occur at a uniform rate around the circumference of the cervix. The process of metaplasia itself is multifocal, developing both as areas of metaplasia adjacent to the original squamous tissue and as discrete islands within the columnar tissue (Figure 4–6). The many metaplastic foci gradually widen, coalesce, and eventually join the peripheral component.

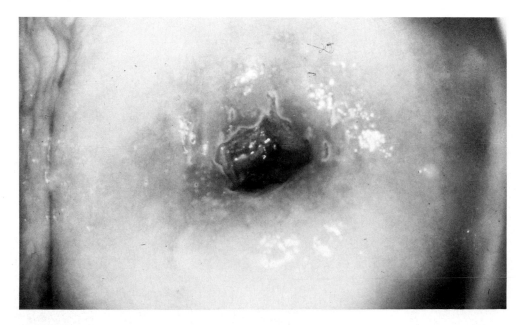

Figure 4-2. Colpophotograph of normal transformation zone. Note the physiologic squamocolumnar junction and gland openings.

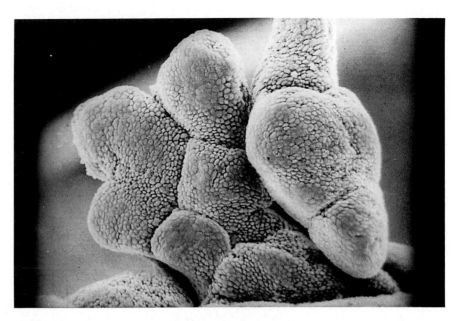

Figure 4-3. Scanning electron micrograph of columnar epithelium undergoing beginning metaplasia. Note the blunting in the tips of some of the villi. *(Reprinted with permission from* The Cervix *by J Jordan and A Singer.)*

HISTOLOGY OF THE TRANSFORMATION ZONE

The earliest evidence of squamous metaplasia in the TZ is "reserve cell hyperplasia," which is the development of a single layer of cuboidal cells beneath the native columnar mucinous cells (Figure 4-7). The precise source of these reserve (or progenitor) cells has been a controversial subject, but recent immunocytochemical studies demonstrating cytokeratins in reserve cells suggest an epithelial origin. Ultrastructurally, these cells also contain numerous mitochondria, free ribosomes, and surface microvilli; they are attached by desmosomes to one another and to adjacent columnar cells.

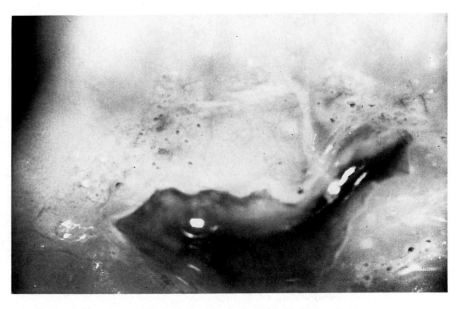

Figure 4-4. Colpophotograph of normal transformation zone with gland openings.

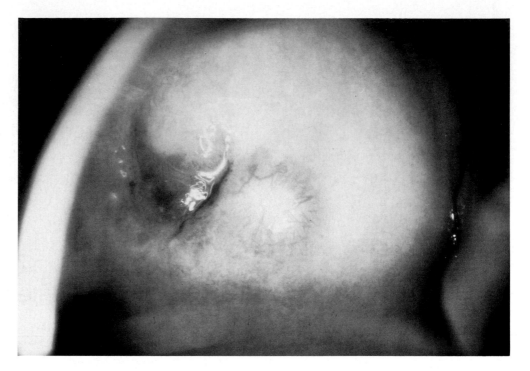

Figure 4-5. Colpophotograph of transformation zone with Nabothian cyst. Note the large dichotomizing blood vessels.

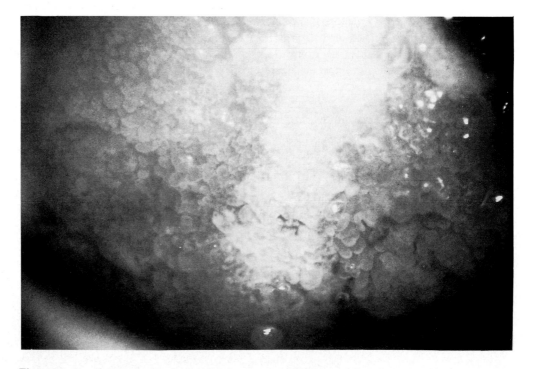

Figure 4-6. Colpophotograph of columnar epithelium with an island of villi beginning the metaplastic process.

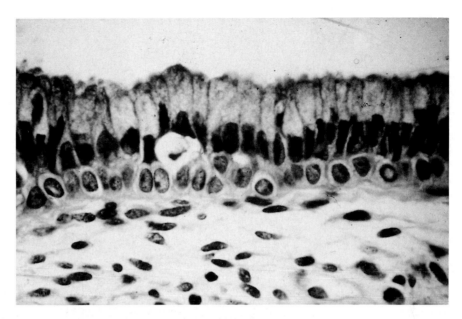

Figure 4-7. Biopsy of columnar epithelium with a single layer of reserve cells. *(Reprinted with permission from* Basic and Advanced Laser Surgery in Gynecology, *by MS Baggish.)*

Progression of squamous metaplasia within the TZ consists of proliferation of reserve cells, thus increasing the number of epithelial cell layers (Figure 4-8). The native columnar cells are lifted by the underlying reserve cells and are ultimately sloughed from the surface (Figure 4-9). The extent of the metaplastic process varies from area to area so that columnar cells, singly or in glandular clusters, may be identified within metaplastic mucosa. The proliferating reserve cells assume squamous characteristics but remain immature. Thus, they have large active nuclei, are often associated with a high mitotic index, and have dense cytoplasm that lacks glycogen (Figure 4-10a, Figure 4-10b). Typical ultrastructural features include numerous cytoplasmic filaments (keratins), prominent desmosomes, and surface microvilli and microridges; the latter best demonstrated by scanning electron microscopy.

Over time (usually a period of years), the squamous epithelium matures. Maturation is characterized by the same features noted in the native squamous epithelium of the cervix as described in Chapter 2. As a result, the fully mature metaplastic epithelium will assume a gross appearance identical to that of the surface of the exocervix except for the possible presence of residual gland openings, Nabothian cysts, and islands of original columnar epithelium (Figure 4-11).

CYTOLOGY OF THE TRANSFORMATION ZONE

In addition to squamous and columnar cells (described in Chapter 2), cytologic smears of the TZ may contain a variety of squamous metaplastic elements. Reserve cells are small, oval to round cells with a fairly high nuclear:cytoplasmic ratio. The nucleus, variably located in the cell, has finely dispersed chromatin whereas the cytoplasm often contains delicate vacuoles (Figure 4-12). The cells of immature squamous metaplasia are larger than reserve cells and their cytoplasm is variable. In some cells it is uniformly dense, but in others the perinuclear zone is less dense than the peripheral cytoplasm (Figure 4-13). The junction of these two zones may be demarcated by a thin filament. Mature squamous metaplastic cells vary in shape from round to polygonal; their cytoplasm also varies, resembling either that of immature metaplastic cells or intermediate

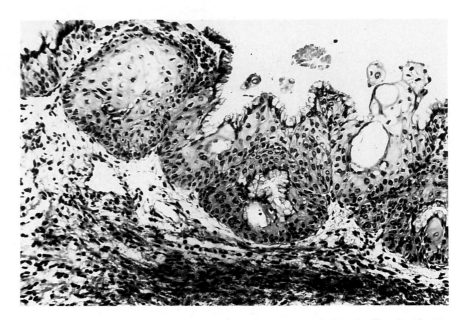

Figure 4-8.   Biopsy showing multiple layers of endocervical immature squamous cells lifting off the original columnar cells.

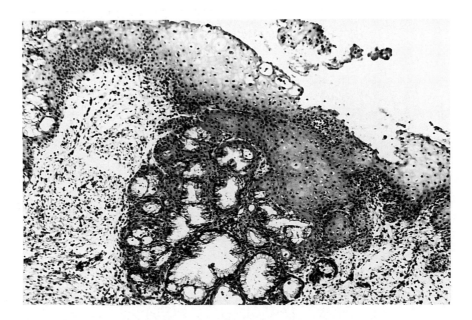

Figure 4-9.   Biopsy showing advanced squamous metaplasia on mucosa. Remnants of columnar epithelium are present on the surface of the mucosa. The underlying endocervical invaginations show much less metaplasia.

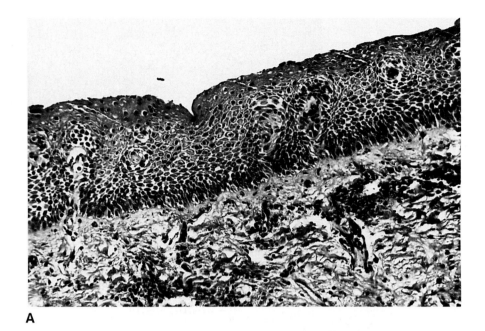

A

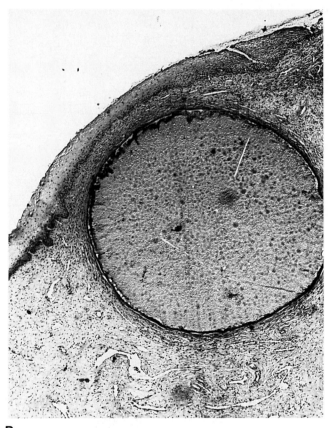

B

Figure 4-10. A. Advanced immature squamous metaplasia. The cytoplasm is dark staining due to the lack of glycogen. No surface glandular cells remain. **B.** Nabothian cyst in the cervical stroma beneath a well-glycogenated, fully mature squamous metaplastic mucosa.

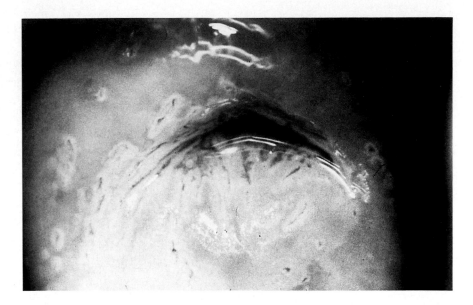

Figure 4-11. Colpophotograph of mature transformation zone with multiple gland openings.

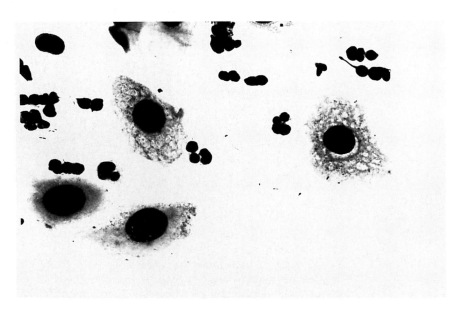

Figure 4-12. Cytosmear of immature squamous metaplasia. Note the cytoplasmic vacuolization.

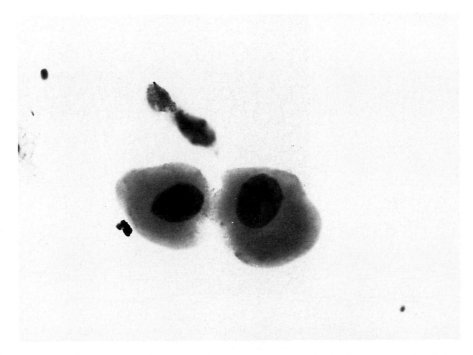

Figure 4-13. Cytosmear of immature squamous metaplasia demonstrating increased nuclear:cytoplasmic ratio.

squamous cells. The nuclei of both immature and mature squamous metaplastic cells have finely granular chromatin, but the nuclear:cytoplasmic ratio is higher in the immature metaplastic cells.

COLPOSCOPY OF THE TRANSFORMATION ZONE

The earliest colposcopic changes of metaplasia involve loss of transluscency at the tips of the villi of columnar epithelium, along with increased demarcation of vascular structures. The tips of the villi stand out as individual opaque areas against a background of red. The red color is created by the columnar tissue that remains within the clefts between the villi (Figure 4-14). After acetic acid is applied, immature squamous metaplastic epithelium becomes more opaque than original squamous epithelium, possibly as the result of the increased nuclear:cytoplasmic ratio exhibited by immature squamous cells. Immature metaplastic epithelium can be difficult to distinguish from cervical intraepithelial neoplasia (CIN) (Figure 4-15). Immature metaplastic tissue is non-glycogenated and is characteristically iodine negative. As a result, staining techniques are not adequate to distinguish early metaplastic tissue from dysplastic tissue. The colposcopic picture can be variable according to the extent of metaplasia. Sometimes only a few tongues can be identified within the columnar epithelium. Alternatively, the original columnar epithelium can be almost completely covered by the metaplastic squamous tissue (Figure 4-16).

As the metaplastic process develops and the villi fuse, the colposcopic picture will change. Although individual opaque villi appear fused, minute humps present on the tissue surface represent the tips of the old villi (Figure 4-17). This tissue is not stained by iodine. As the process approaches complete maturation, a smooth surface is produced. The vascular supply becomes similar to that of the original squamous epithelium as the vessels of the columnar papillae are pushed down with the development of the

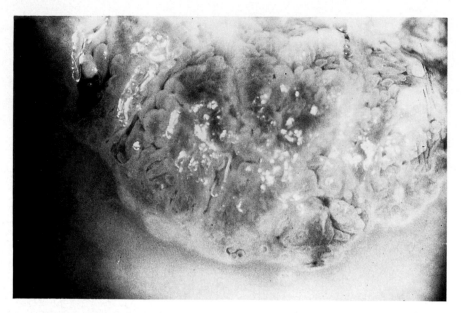

Figure 4-14. Colpophotograph of posterior lip of the cervix showing areas of fused villi in an early metaplastic process and areas of original columnar epithelium that are not participating in the process.

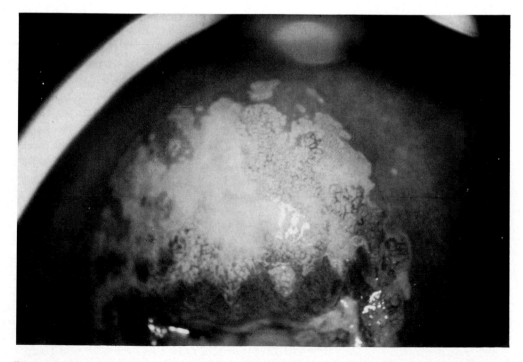

Figure 4-15. Colpophotograph of the anterior lip of the cervix after the application of acetic acid. Note the development of both aceto-white and mosaic changes.

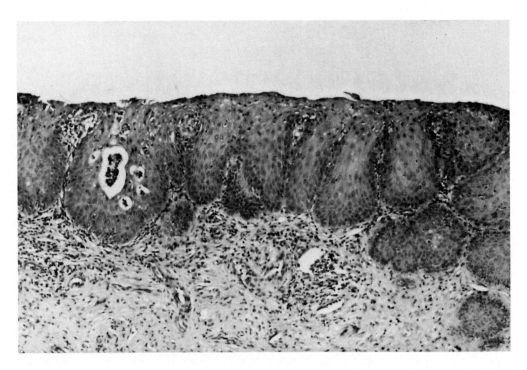

Figure 4-16. Biopsy of the mosaic area seen in Figure 4-15. The epithelium is metaplastic. Note the vessels coming up into the areas of metaplasia, forming the mosaic colposcopic appearance.

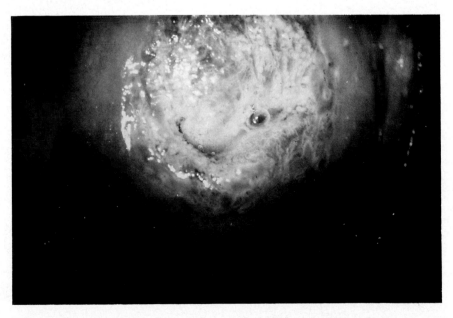

Figure 4-17. Colpophotograph of developing transformation zone with the columnar epithelium almost completely replaced with metaplastic epithelium.

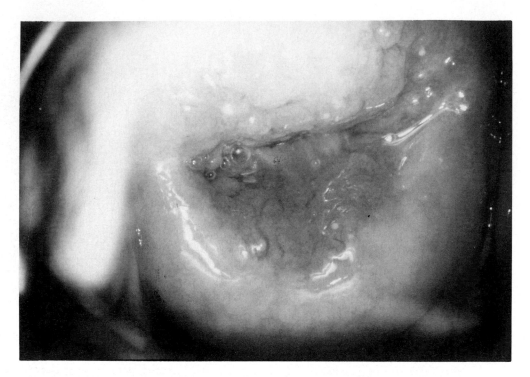

Figure 4-18. Colpophotograph showing large terminal vessel in an area of active metaplasia. Note that these vessels do divide.

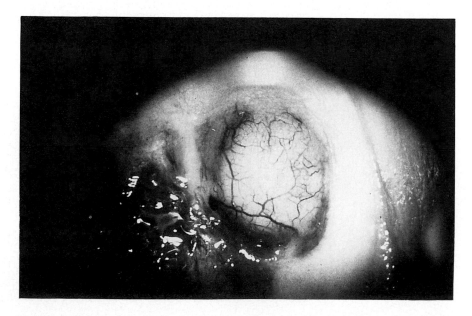

Figure 4-19. Colpophotograph of the anterior lip of the cervix with a large Nabothian cyst. The characteristic vasculature of this structure is obvious.

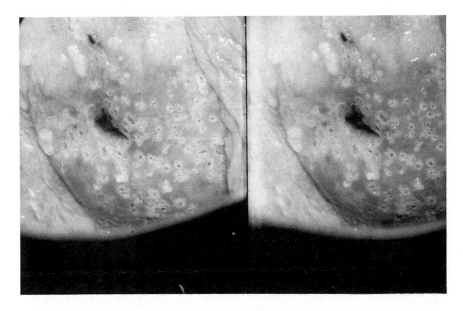

Figure 4-20. Colpophotograph of cervix of a patient exposed in utero to diethylstilbestrol. Note the numerous "white rimmed" glands covering the exocervix.

new squamous metaplastic epithelium. Mature metaplastic tissue exhibits both network and hairpin capillaries of varying number and pattern. In the normal mature TZ, a terminal vessel running parallel with the tissue surface may commonly be seen (Figure 4-18). It is strikingly large and divides dichotomously into a network of delicate capillaries with normal or even increased intercapillary distances. Such vessels are frequently associated with Nabothian cysts (Figure 4-19).

Gland openings colposcopically appear as dark red craters encircled by a dense white border (Figure 4-20). Nabothian cysts are yellowish and transluscent and are elevated above the level of the surrounding epithelium. The mature metaplastic squamous epithelium colposcopically can only be identified by the presence of columnar remnants (islands of columnar cells, Nabothian cysts, and gland openings). These remnants serve to define the distal margin of the TZ, the original border between the native squamous and the metaplastic squamous epithelium.

Chapter 5 | Atypical Transformation Zone

ATYPICAL COLPOSCOPIC TISSUE PATTERNS

In the presence of oncogenic stimuli, the columnar epithelilum in the transformation zone (TZ) undergoes atypical squamous metaplasia. The precise mechanisms of neoplastic cellular transformation are not fully elucidated, but the morphologic consequence is a diminution or loss of control mechanisms regulating cellular proliferation. Thus, the transformed metaplastic epithelium starts to grow in buds or blocks, completely filling the clefts and folds of the endocervix within the TZ. As abnormal proliferation progresses, the neoplastic cells release a factor, called the tumor angiogenesis factor (TAF), that progresses proliferation of adjacent capillaries to insure the nutrition of the abnormal epithelium (Figure 5-1). As a result, the subepithelial vascular network undergoes profound alteration, as determined by examination of histochemical vascular preparations and by colposcopic observations.

Depending on the precise point in time during the metaplastic process at which neoplastic transformation occurs, the vascular capillary network will become tortuous and compressed vertically to variable degrees by the neoplastic epithelium. Transformation early in metaplasia will permit vessels to extend either close to the surface, producing the colposcopic pattern of punctation (Figure 5-2, Figure 5-3), or halfway up the epithelium, producing a basket weave structure around the epithelium, resulting in the colposcopic appearance called mosaicism (Figure 5-4, Figure 5-5, Figure 5-6, Color Plates 5, 6, 7a, 7b). If neoplastic alteration in the cell occurs late in metaplasia after all of the capillaries have been pushed down from the papillae, the colposcopic appearance is termed aceto-white epithelium (Figure 5-7, Figure 5-8, Figure 5-9). Aceto-white epithelium can be appreciated only after the application of acetic acid. The whitening of the epithelium is a transient phenomenon that is seen in areas of increased nuclear density. If the abnormal epithelium produces keratin on its surface, a leukoplakic lesion will develop that can be seen with the naked eye in a good light; it does not require magnification (see Figure 1-3). If there is neoangiogenesis, new capillaries will be formed, producing what are called atypical blood vessels (Figure 5-10, Color Plate 8).

Thus, a TZ is said to be abnormal if any of the following are seen:

1. Aceto-white epithelium.
2. Punctation.
3. Mosaic.
4. Leukoplakia (hyperkeratosis).
5. Abnormal blood vessels.

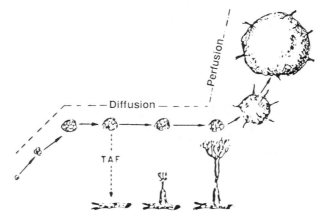

Illustration of the concept that most solid tumors may exist early as tiny cell populations living by simple diffusion in the extracellular space. (Further growth requires vascularization and the tumor then maintains itself by perfusion.) Tumor angiogenesis factor (TAF) may be the mediator of neovascularization.

Figure 5-1.   Diagram illustrating the mechanism of action of tumor angiogenesis factor. *(Reprinted with permission from* The New England Journal of Medicine, *by J. Folkman.)*

An atypical TZ is, therefore, readily identified colposcopically. The five atypical colposcopic tissue patterns noted above may occur singly or in combination. They may be unifocal or multifocal, and they are usually sharply delineated from the surrounding normal tissue.

With the exception of leukoplakia, none of these lesions of the atypical TZ can be seen with the naked eye prior to the application of acetic acid. Areas of punctation, mosaic, and abnormal blood vessels, however, can be seen through the colposcope with magnification utilizing a green filter but without acetic acid if the mucous membrane is observed through a film of saline (*see* Figure 5-4).

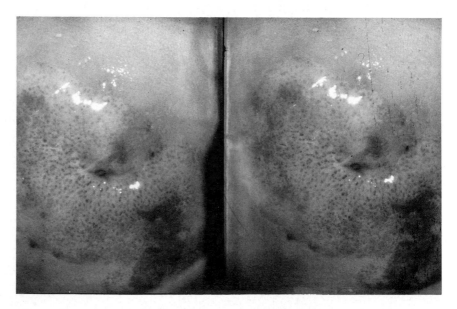

Figure 5-2.   Colpophotograph of punctation with increased intercapillary distances.

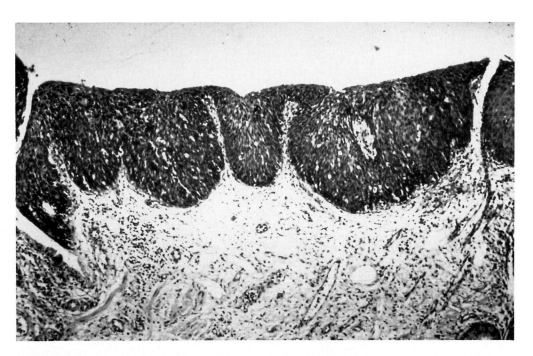

Figure 5-3. Biopsy of Figure 5-2 showing cervical intraepithelial neoplasia III. Vessels penetrate the abnormal epithelium producing the punctate appearance.

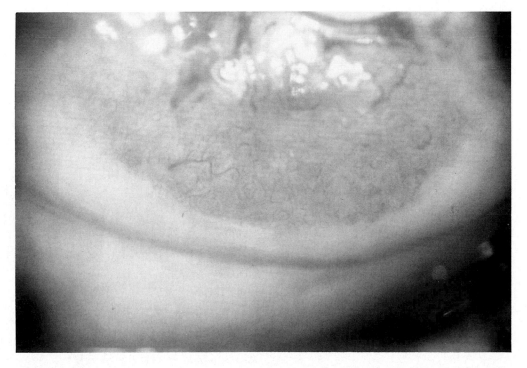

Figure 5-4. Colpophotograph of posterior lip of the cervix viewed through a thin film of saline. Vessels are present surrounding blocks of epithelium.

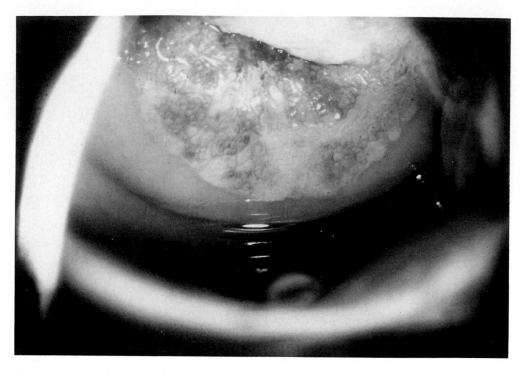

Figure 5-5. Colpophotograph after the application of acetic acid. The mosaicism is apparent.

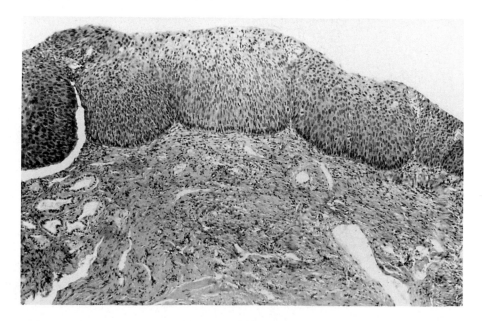

Figure 5-6. Photomicrograph of biopsy taken from the area shown in Figure 5-5. Note that vessels only penetrate half of the thickness of the epithelium. Diagnosis: CIN II to III.

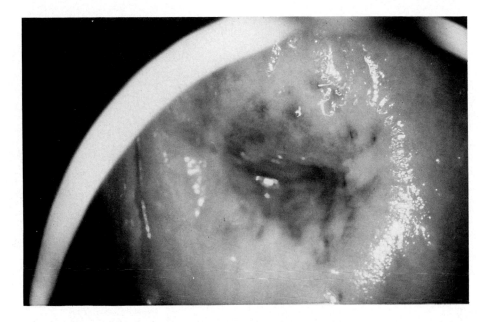

Figure 5-7. Colpophotograph of patient with abnormal cytosmear prior to the application of acetic acid. No obvious aberrations are seen.

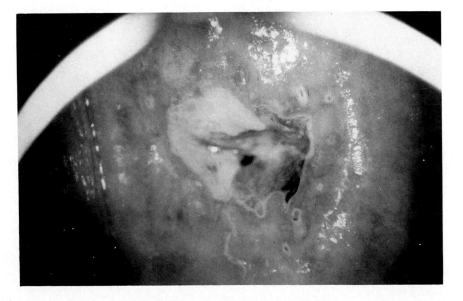

Figure 5-8. Colpophotograph of the cervix shown in Figure 5-7 after the application of acetic acid. Note the sharply demarcated aceto-white lesion seen at 9 to 12 o'clock.

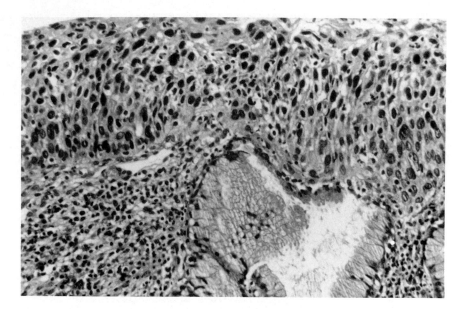

Figure 5-9. Photomicrograph of biopsy of the aceto-white lesion in Figure 5-8 at 12 o'clock. Note that dysplastic cells occupy the full thickness of the epithelium (CIN III).

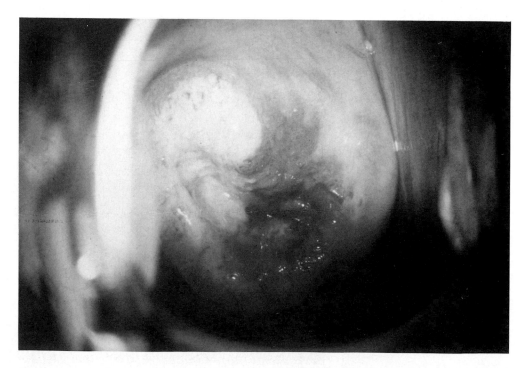

Figure 5-10. Colpophotograph of cervix with invasive carcinoma. Note atypical blood vessels between 10 and 12 o'clock.

It should be recognized that any condition that causes increased cellular division, abnormal cellular metabolism or increased vascularization can cause these atypicalities. Thus, infection, inflammation, regeneration, repair, and pregnancy, as well as neoplasia, can result in the development of an atypical TZ. Neoplasia, however, produces the most striking changes and can be delineated colposcopically from the most benign conditions. It should be noted that some of these changes seen in the cervical TZ can also be appreciated on other mucous membranes, such as those of the vagina, vulva, anus, and oral cavity.

Aceto-White Epithelium

Aceto-white epithelium is the most frequent abnormality in the atypical TZ. It usually has a flat, smooth surface that is level with the surrounding tissue and does not contain visible terminal vessels. As noted earlier, the area usually cannot be distinguished from normal tissue without colposcopic magnification aided by the application of either saline plus the use of the green filter, or by the application of acetic acid (Figure 5–11, Figure 5–12). The more severe aceto-white lesions, however, may be suspected at initial inspection at the time of colposcopy by the presence of a slightly opaque surface on the cervical mucosa. Whiteness, presumably, is related to the nuclear predominance in the atypical cells, the reversal of the nuclear:cytoplasmic ratio, the increase in epithelial cell numbers, the abnormally large amounts of DNA, and the increased cytoplasmic density in the altered squamous cells.

There are many theories why the epithelium turns white with the application of acetic acid. Of interest, in none of Hinselmann's early writings does he explain either the reason for his choice of acetic acid or his concept of the pathogenesis of the aceto-white change. A common theory in the past has been that because of the presence of large amounts of atypical nuclear and cytoplasmic protein in the abnormal cells, acetic acid causes denaturing and congealing of the protein, thus inhibiting the transmission of light. If this were true, however, the change induced by acetic acid would not be transient because denatured protein cannot rearrange itself back to normal after the effect of acetic acid wears off. A more plausible explanation proposes that acetic acid induces an osmotic change in cervical tissue, resulting in hypertonicity of the extracellular space. Water exits from the cell, and the cellular membrane collapses around the nucleus. The concentration of nuclear DNA per unit area is increased, thus inhibiting the transmission of the colposcopic light and producing the intense white change. As the acetic acid dissipates from the tissue and its effect wears off, water returns to the cell, the cell membrane expands, and the whiteness disappears. Because the whitening phenomenon is transient, it can be repeated by the reapplication of acetic acid.

The degree of whiteness is a reflection of the number, size, and DNA concentration of the abnormal cells: the more intense the whiteness, the more abnormal the underlying epithelium. This intensity can be measured precisely by placing a filter in the eyepiece of the colposcope and determining the intensity in Angstrom units. In clinical practice, however, the colposcopist tends to grade the intensity subjectively in terms of white, whiter, and whitest. In addition to the intensity of the whiteness, the speed with which it occurs, its duration, and the rapidness of its disappearance also correlate with the underlying histopathology. The more rapid the appearance of the change, the longer its duration, and the slower its disappearance, the more severe is the abnormality in the cells. Another variable feature of aceto-white epithelium is the characteristic of its margin with the surrounding normal epithelium: the sharper the border the more abnormal the tissue. The reason for this well-defined interface is not completely known; both immunologic factors and possible epithelial hormonal factors have been implicated in its development.

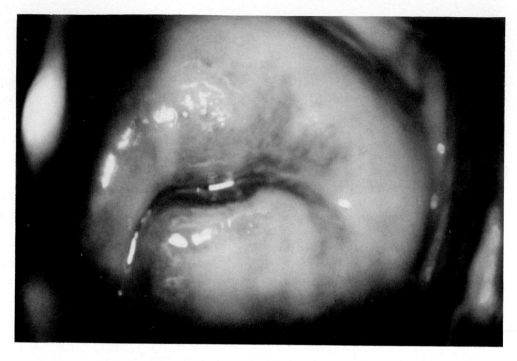

Figure 5-11. Colpophotograph of cervix after the application of saline. Note the innocuous appearance of the cervix.

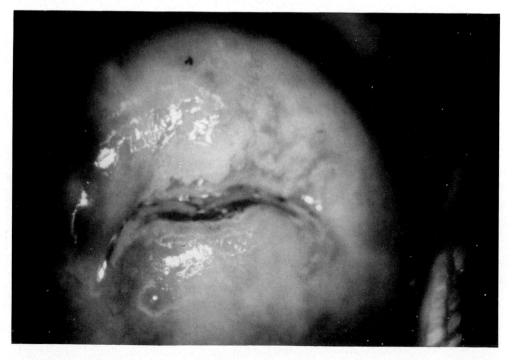

Figure 5-12. Colpophotograph of cervix shown in Figure 5-11, after the application of acetic acid. Note aceto-white lesion at 12 o'clock. (Histology: CIN I to II.)

Wespi has suggested that the colposcopic image of the uterine cervix following acetic acid can be enhanced by the application of a 0.5% salicylic acid alcohol solution, which intensifies the acetic acid whiteness (Figures 5-13, 5-14, 5-15, 5-16, 5-17). Immature squamous epithelium will show a more intense opaque-whitish appearance while the glandular epithelium increases its reddish tinge. Thus, the border between squamous and glandular epithelium becomes more distinct and shows more contrast—features that are beneficial for the colposcopist. The appearance of the mature squamous epithelium is not influenced by salicylic acid alcohol.

Punctation and Mosaic Structures

As noted above, during atypical metaplasia as the result of the influence of TAF, changes in the capillaries of the columnar epithelium papillae occur in conjunction with the development of the blocks or buds of abnormal cells. The vascular network within each villus persists and undergoes marked proliferation. The central vascular network of these remaining stromal papillae feature blood vessel loops that extend close to the surface of the overlying epithelium or halfway up the thickness of the epithelium. Punctation and mosaic patterns are reflections of this abnormal developmental process.

Progression of atypical metaplasia is characterized by increased proliferation activity of the squamous epithelium within the clefts and lateral compression of the stromal papillae. The hairpin or loop vessels within the papillae may undergo dilatation and proliferation near the surface or may form ramifications around buds of atypical epithelium. In the first instance, capillaries form a stipple pattern and the lesion appears colposcopically as punctation; in the second case, a mosaic structure is observed. Because the process of development of the mosaic and the punctation patterns from original columnar epithelium are basically very similar, both tissue types frequently are found in the same lesion (Figure 5-18, see Color Plate 7b).

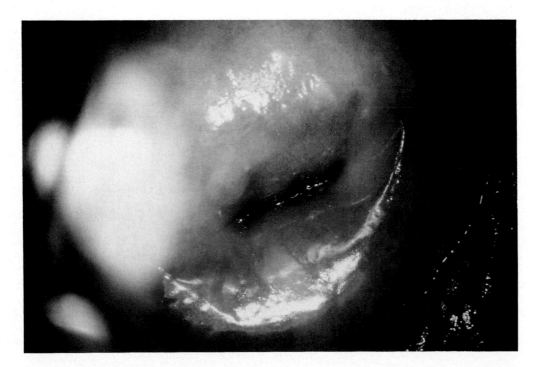

Figure 5-13. Colpophotograph of the cervix after the application of saline. Close observation reveals a subtle vascular change suggestive of a mosaic pattern on the anterior lip. (Compare with Figure 5-4.)

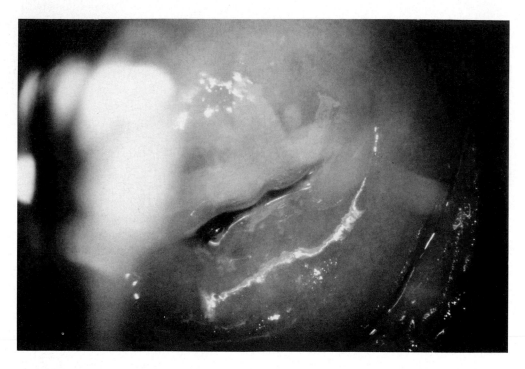

Figure 5-14.   Cervix in Figure 5-13 after the application of acetic acid. An abnormal transformation zone is now evident on the anterior lip, suggestive of a mosaic pattern.

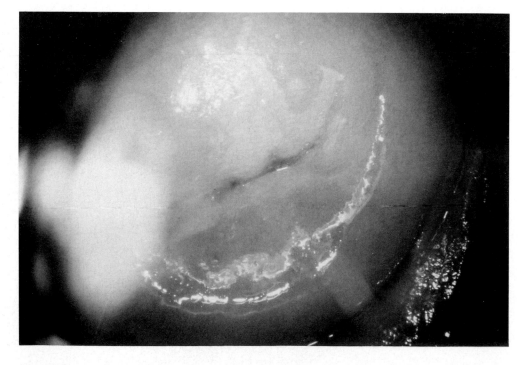

Figure 5-15.   Cervix in Figure 5-14 after the application of 0.5% salicylic alcohol. Note that the mosaic structure is less obvious and that the aceto-white appearance is intensified.

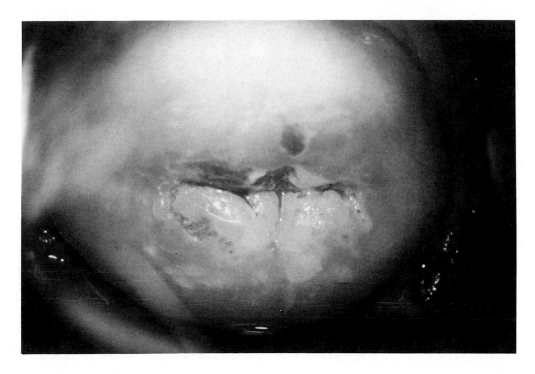

Figure 5-16. Cervix after the application of acetic acid. Note the aceto-white change at 1 o'clock and at 4 to 9 o'clock.

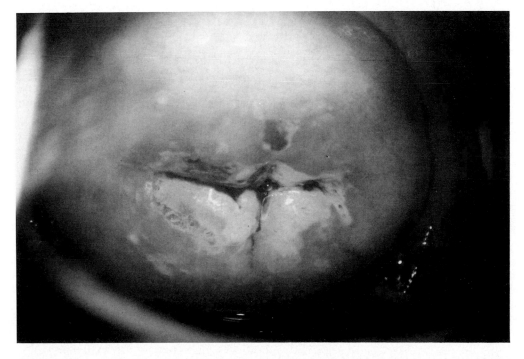

Figure 5-17. Cervix shown in Figure 5-16, after the application of 0.5% salicylic alcohol. Note that portions of the aceto-white lesion have been enhanced.

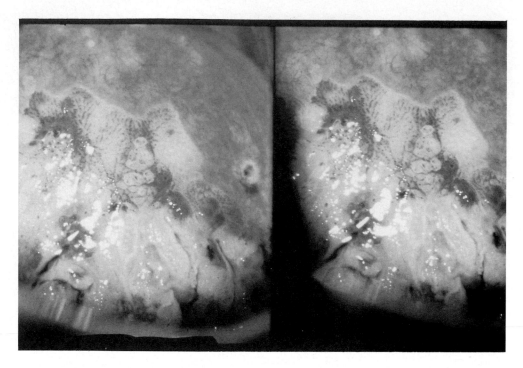

Figure 5-18. Cervix after the application of acetic acid. Note that the lesion contains both mosaic pattern and punctation.

Colposcopically, punctation and mosaic terminal vessels may show wide variations in size, shape, arrangement, and intercapillary distance depending on the degree of the associated histologic atypia. Punctation may be delicate and regular with normal intercapillary distances. Alternatively, capillary loops may appear markedly dilated and tortuous with increased distance between individual vessels. Mosaic terminal vessels also may be fine or coarse and regular or irregular; such vessels may outline fields that are small, large, round, polygonal, or pleomorphic in nature. Increased intercapillary distance and irregularity of mosaic tiles is caused by a disordered compression and disappearance of some stromal papillae by the rapidly proliferating typical epithelium. In general, the more irregular the mosaic pattern, the more significant is the histologic lesion (Table 5-1).

Squamous metaplasia without any apparent malignant potential can also exhibit punctation and mosaic patterns. The mosaic in many places consists of delicate terminal capillaries coursing around small gland openings. There are certain characteristics that indicate that the punctation and mosaic patterns are likely to be innocuous; the color

TABLE 5-1. INTERCAPILLARY DISTANCE AND HISTOLOGIC DIAGNOSIS

Histologic Diagnosis	Intercapillary Distance > 300 μ (%)
Benign lesions	1.8
Dysplasia	14.6
Carcinoma in situ	57.1
Early invasive carcinoma	76.9
Invasive carcinoma	85.5

Normal mucous membrane of cervix = 50 to 250 μ.
After Kolstad. (See Bibliography.)

of the epithelium is normal, the surface is smooth and level with the adjacent original squamous epithelium, and the border of the lesion is indefinite or obscure. The intercapillary distance is essentially normal (Figure 5–19). Significant punctation will generally be found within a well-demarcated area of aceto-white epithelium (*see* Figure 5–2, Figure 5–18). Punctation, without an associated white lesion, occurs in normal, atrophic, or inflammatory states and has only minor significance. Thus, to be significant, mosaic and punctate vessels must be seen within areas of sharply demarcated aceto-white epithelium and have some degree of vascular dilatation and change in their intercapillary distance.

Leukoplakia

As already noted, leukoplakia can be diagnosed without colposcopy. It can be seen prior to the application of acetic acid and with the naked eye (Figure 5–20). Histologically, leukoplakia merely shows hyperkeratosis or parakeratosis (Figure 5–21). Keratosis appears as a clearly demarcated, white area with an irregular border. The white appearance is due to reflection of incident light by a dense layer of superficial cornified epithelium. Because of its considerable opacity, keratosis obscures the underlying vascular structure and prevents analysis of the underlying tissue structures. Localization of the keratosis is important. When it overlies normal squamous epithelium, it is usually of minor significance, frequently being evidence of human papilloma viral (HPV) infection. When present within the TZ, especially when surrounded by white epithelium, mosaic or punctation, it has greater significance. The significance, however, usually lies not within the keratotic area but in the adjacent tissue.

Atypical Blood Vessels

As the intraepithelial lesion develops it may reach a stage where it will remain dormant for years. With the release of TAF, new capillaries will be stimulated to develop. These

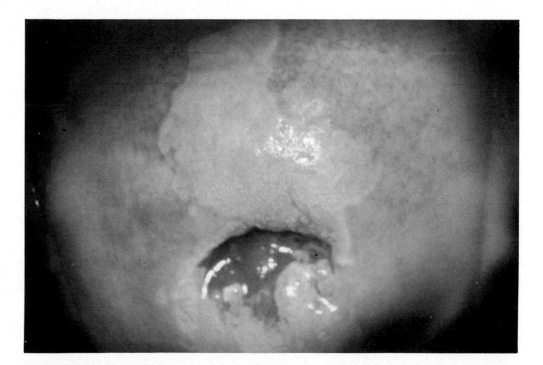

Figure 5–19. Cervix after the application of acetic acid, showing grade I mosaic pattern with normal intercapillary distances. On biopsy this area is immature squamous metaplasia.

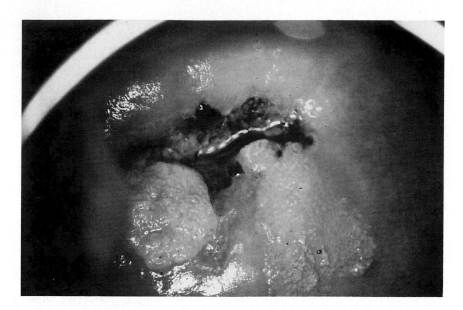

Figure 5-20. Cervix prior to the application of acetic acid. Note the large area of leukoplakia on the posterior lip of the cervix.

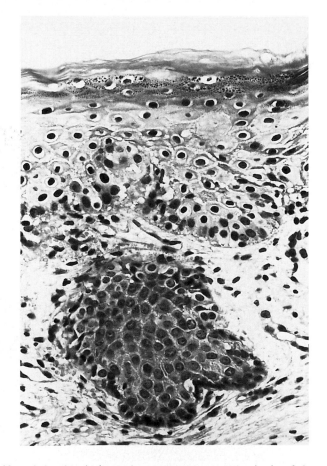

Figure 5-21. Keratinization in immature squamous metaplasia of the cervix. At the bottom of the photograph, an endocervical invagination is replaced by immature squamous cells. On the surface, the upper layers of metaplastic squamous cells contain keratohyaline granules.

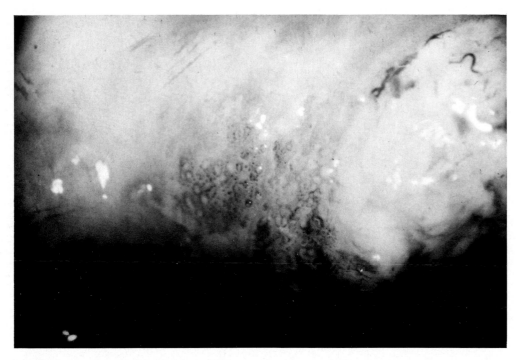

Figure 5-22. Cervix with invasive cancer on the anterior lip. Note prominent atypical blood vessels on the left.

are usually underneath the surface of the epithelium and parallel to it. They are usually nondividing vessels and have a variety of shapes and appearances as already noted. These vessels do not arborize as do the normal vessels of the squamous epithelium. Because they are not normal they are called atypical blood vessels. With their appearance the increase in intercapillary distance may at first be somewhat decreased; as the tumor expands and compresses, the intercapillary distance will increase.

These atypical vessels may appear colposcopically as a coarse meshwork enclosing irregular avascular fields, as irregular branch patterns showing no steady decrease in the diameter of terminal branches, or as a single vessel with sharp, irregular bends, "spaghetti" forms, and various other appearances. They may be reminiscent of commas or corkscrews and are correlated with the degree of malignant histologic change (Figure 5-22, Color Plates 2, 16). Vessels of this nature are most often colposcopic indicators of microinvasive disease or invasive carcinoma (Table 5-2). Figure 5-23 is the allogram of the development of both the typical and atypical transformation zone.

TABLE 5-2. ATYPICAL VESSELS AND HISTOLOGIC DIAGNOSIS

Histologic Diagnosis	Atypical Vessels (%)
Benign lesion	0.6
Dysplasia	0.7
Carcinoma in situ	16.7
Early invasive carcinoma	76.9
Invasive carcinoma	96.6

After Kolstad. (See Bibliography.)

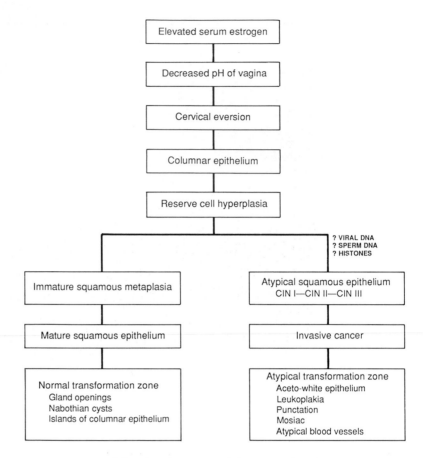

Figure 5-23. Allogram of the development of the normal and abnormal transformation zone.

GRADING OF COLPOSCOPIC LESIONS

Although the atypical TZ identifies the site and extent of major intraepithelial neoplastic changes as well as true invasion, many atypical TZs demonstrate only minor histologic disturbances in cervical epithelia and are of no apparent clinical significance. All things being equal, the more abnormal the colposcopic appearance the greater the histologic abnormalities. It is possible for an experienced colposcopist to differentiate the various forms of intraepithelial neoplasia from early invasive cancer on the basis of the colposcopic features. The features that are utilized are those of color, surface contour, vascular patterns, intercapillary distances, and the overall grade of the abnormality of the lesion.

The quality of the abnormal colposcopic lesion, as already noted, depends on the degree of whiteness of the epithelium, the rapidity with which the whiteness occurs, the nature of the surface contour, whether flat or irregular, the fineness or coarseness of the caliber of the punctate vessels and their intercapillary distances, the irregularity and pleomorphism of the mosaic pattern, and the presence or absence of atypical blood vessels (Table 5-3). The intercapillary distance is an extremely important indicator of the seriousness or severity of the atypicality of the colposcopic lesion. As shown by Kolstad, as the intercapillary distance increases above 300 μ (see Table 5-1), the more serious intraepithelial neoplastic lesions are likely to occur. The only place where this is less likely to happen is at the moment of microinvasion when new capillaries are pro-

TABLE 5-3. DIAGNOSTIC PRINCIPLES OF COLPOSCOPY

Surface contour
Margin of lesion
Whiteness of lesion
Speed of aceto-white change
Vascular patterns and intercapillary distance
Atypical blood vessels

duced, and there may be a slight decrease in the intercapillary distance.

Interpretation of the atypical transformation zone based on these various features is seen in Table 5–4.

Grade I Lesions

The color tone of a grade I lesion is judged as normal or slightly whiter than normal, especially when viewed through the green filter. The surface is smooth; the border of the lesion tends to be somewhat diffuse (Figure 5–24a, Figure 5–24b, Color Plate 10a, Color Plate 10b). The lesion takes a moderate length of time to develop, stays a very short time, and disappears rapidly. If there are any vascular changes present, it is characterized by a fine or regular punctate appearance, mosaic appearance, or both; there is no increase in the intercapillary distances. This type of lesion may be seen in anything from HPV infection, pregnancy, metaplasia, inflammation, regeneration, and repair.

Grade II Lesions

A grade II lesion has a more intense whiteness and appears in what one might call a normal time span. It tends to stay for several minutes and then disappears with average speed. It usually has a sharp border dividing it from the surrounding normal epithelium (Figure 5–25, Color Plate 11). There is usually some vascular pattern in the form of an irregular punctation or mosaic with a slight increase in the intercapillary distances. This may represent mild to moderate intraepithelial neoplastic changes as well as HPV infection.

Grade III Lesions

Grade III lesions have a clearcut elevation of the surface pattern. The border of the grade III lesion is sharp and distinct (Figure 5–26). There is a marked intensity to the whiteness of the epithelium. The lesion develops rapidly, stays a long time, and slowly fades away (Figures 5–27, 5–28, 5–29, Color Plate 12). If punctation or mosaic structures are

TABLE 5-4. GRADING COLPOSCOPIC LESIONS

Grade	Surface	Margin	Color	Time	Vessels	Pathology
I	Flat	Indistinct	White	Slow/short	Fine: normal ICD	Insignificant infection, repair HPV
II	Flat	Distinct	Whiter	Average/average	Dilated Pn, mosaic, slight ↑ ICD	Significant HPV, CIN I, CIN II
III	Raised	Sharp	Whitest	Fast/long	Coarse: marked ↑ ICD, atypical BV	Highly significant CIN III, microinvasion-invasion

BV = blood vessel; CIN = cervical intraepithelial neoplasia; HPV = human papilloma virus; ICD = intercapillary distance; Pn = punctation.

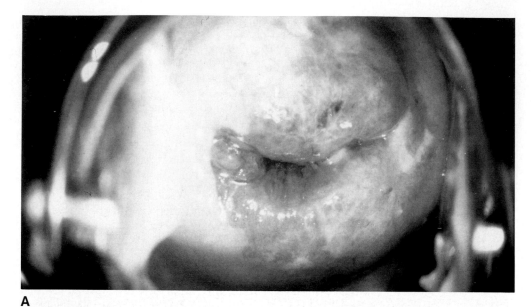

A

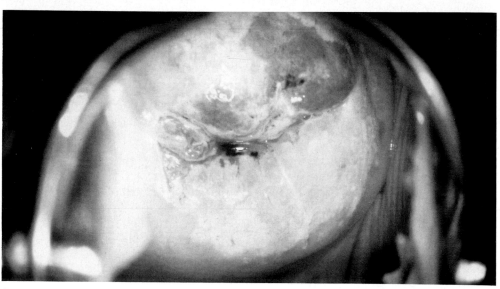

B

Figure 5-24.   A. Cervix prior to the application of acetic acid. No abnormalities noted. **B.** Cervix after the application of acetic acid. Note the grade I aceto-white change from 4 to 8 o'clock. The periphery of the lesion at 4 to 5 o'clock has an innocuous mosaic structure. Biopsy revealed HPV-related changes and metaplasia.

present, the intercapillary distances are usually increased (Figure 5–30). Frequently in this type of lesion, when the acid is applied, the epithelium may roll up like wet cigarette paper, indicating a loss of the intercellular bonds. There may be a loss of surface epithelium and ulceration; in the invasive lesion, atypical blood vessels may be bizarre. The grade III lesion may represent the more severe intraepithelial neoplastic lesions, microinvasion, or invasive disease (*see* Chapter 6).

Colposcopic gradings in general correlate with the underlying histology. The greater the histologic abnormality the more pronounced are the colposcopic changes.

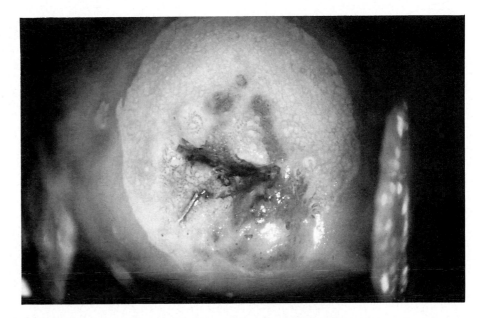

Figure 5-25. Cervix after the application of acetic acid. There is a grade II mosaic structure surrounding the os. The border is sharp. The tiles are somewhat irregular with slight increase in the intercapillary distances. Biopsy revealed CIN II.

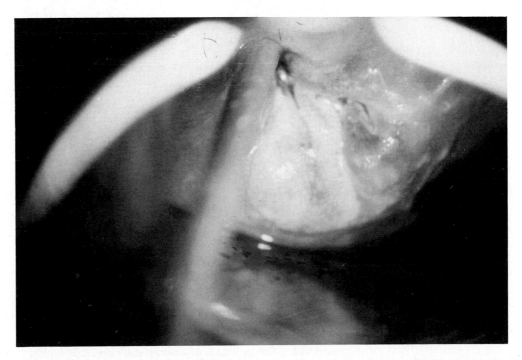

Figure 5-26. Cervix after the application of acetic acid. There is a sharply delineated aceto-white lesion on the posterior lip of the cervix. Biopsy revealed CIN III.

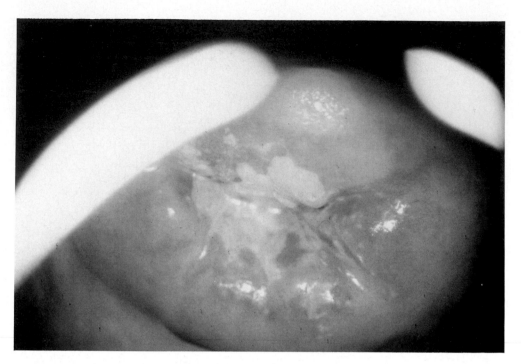

Figure 5–27.   Cervix with a grade III aceto-white change at 12 o'clock after the application of acetic acid. There is a grade I change at 6 to 8 o'clock. The anterior lesion is intensely white and sharply delineated. Biopsy at 12 o'clock showed CIN III; biopsy at 7 o'clock showed HPV changes.

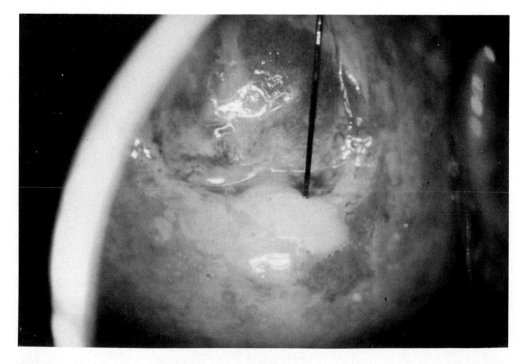

Figure 5–28.   Posterior lip of the cervix after acetic acid. There is a raised, intensely white grade III lesion at 5 to 6 o'clock. This is superimposed on a grade I aceto-white change.

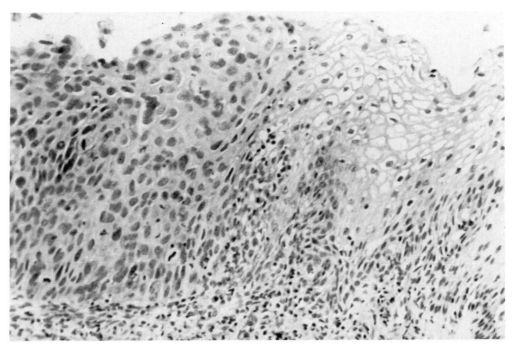

Figure 5-29. Biopsy at the edge of the grade III aceto-white lesion of Figure 5-27. On the left, CIN grade II to III is present and sharply demarcated from an area showing condylomatous features.

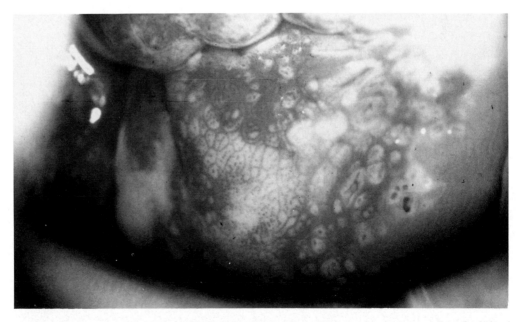

Figure 5-30. Posterior lip of the cervix with a grade III mosaic change at 5 to 6 o'clock and a grade II mosaic change at 6 to 8 o'clock. The tiles at 5 to 6 o'clock are pleomorphic and the vascular channels are dilated and have increased intercapillary distances. The tiles at 6 to 8 o'clock are somewhat more symmetrical and the vascular channels are not as dilated as those at 5 to 6 o'clock. Biopsy at 5 o'clock revealed CIN III; biopsy at 7 o'clock revealed CIN II.

Chapter 6 | Cervical Intraepithelial Neoplasia

Invasive squamous cell carcinoma of the cervix is the end result of a series of progressive in situ dysplastic changes occurring in metaplastic squamous mucosa (Figure 6–1). In the past, this preinvasive phase was divided into separate entities called dysplasia (mild, moderate, and severe) and carcinoma in situ, with the implication that the latter had a greater propensity to invade than the former. Based on a variety of clinical and laboratory studies, both dysplasia and carcinoma in situ are considered parts of a biologic continuum of preinvasive disease that may be termed cervical intraepithelial neoplasia (CIN).

INCIDENCE OF CERVICAL INTRAEPITHELIAL NEOPLASIA

Most authorities agree that CIN is a venereal disease with a long incubation period. A higher relative risk is associated with early sexual experience (by age 17) and with exposure to multiple male partners. Pregnancy by age 17 is also an important discriminating variable. In addition, host factors such as genetic and immunologic makeup, history of sexually transmitted diseases, and smoking are important variables influencing the genesis and clinical expression of CIN. Although the peak in the age specific prevalence of carcinoma in situ occurs in the 30- to 40-year age group, the peak incidence rates occur in the 20- to 30-year-olds. The precursor lesions often occur in teenagers; 30% of women with CIN will first be diagnosed when they are less than 20 years of age. Investigations suggest that approximately 50% of patients with CIN will develop these dysplastic changes within 5 years after the onset of sexual activity.

Clinically, CIN is usually asymptomatic and first is detected in cytosmears. Occasional patients will report retrospectively that they have had bleeding either after coitus or with the insertion and removal of a vaginal tampon or diaphragm. The examiner may note leukoplakia on the cervix or excessive bleeding at the time of taking routine cytology.

COLPOSCOPY AND PATHOLOGY OF CERVICAL INTRAEPITHELIAL NEOPLASIA

Cervical intraepithelial neoplasia, as already noted, includes the entire biologic spectrum of intraepithelial disease that antedates invasive squamous cell carcinoma. Cervical intraepithelial neoplasia can be divided into three grades as follows:

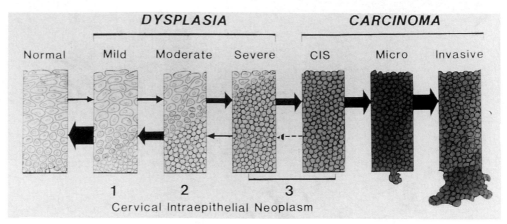

Figure 6-1. Diagram representing the terminology and histologic features of the tissue changes in squamous mucosa from normal to invasive carcinoma.

- CIN I, which is equivalent to mild dysplasia in the old classification.
- CIN II, which is equivalent to moderate dysplasia.
- CIN III, which combines severe dysplasia and carcinoma in situ.

The CIN III designation is particularly useful because it eliminates the biologically false dichotomy between severe dysplasia and in situ carcinoma.

The pathologic diagnosis of CIN requires the recognition of a disordered pattern of squamous cell maturation and significant nuclear atypicality. The major diagnostic criteria of CIN involve the squamous cell nucleus and include increased nuclear chromatin, aberrations of chromatin pattern, and margination of chromatin at the periphery of the nucleus, adjacent to the nuclear membrane (Figure 6–2). The increase in chromatin material results in enhanced basophilic staining and enlargement of the nuclei; thus, the nuclear:cytoplasmic ratio is increased. The abnormal, immature cells

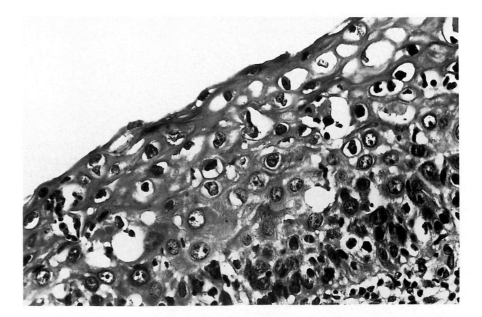

Figure 6-2. High power view of CIN I. At the base, nuclei are enlarged and hyperchromatic. As the dysplastic cells mature, they express cytopathic effects of HPV infection.

continue to be mitotically active; as a result, mitoses, often with abnormal configurations, are noted above the basal zone (Figure 6–3). Cellular density is increased with a subsequently increased number of nuclei per unit area of cervical mucosa (Figure 6–4). Within increasing degrees of severity, CIN is associated with a decrease in cytoplasmic maturation, characterized by a diminution of cytoplasmic glycogen. In most examples of CIN III, glycogen is essentially lost, and the surface cells consist of nuclei surrounded by a thin rim of dark staining cytoplasm (Figure 6–5).

The squamous epithelium showing CIN may become variably thickened (acanthosis), with the occasional development of keratinization at the luminal surface (Figure 6–6). The increased and abnormal proliferation of cells requires increased nutrition and also distorts the subjacent stroma; thus, there are changes in the number and contour of vessels as well as in their intercapillary distances, but these changes are best appreciated by colposcopy (see Chapter 5).

Cervical Intraepithelial Neoplasia I

In CIN I, the cellular changes just described are evident in the lowest third of the mucosa, with maturation above this level (see Figure 6–2). Cytologic smears will reflect this degree of change (Figure 6–7). In CIN I the superficial cells in cytosmears will be relatively normal in size and contain nuclei that are only slightly larger than normal and have only a modest degree of hyperchromasia.

Colposcopically, the lesions of CIN I are nondescript (Figure 6–8a, Figure 6–8b). They are frequently confused with metaplasia, human papilloma viral (HPV) infection, pregnancy, and repair. The aceto-white change usually comes on slowly, lasts a short time, and fades quickly. The lesions are flat and have an opaque to pale white appearance, with margins that tend to be feathery and indistinct. Usually no vascular changes are seen. If there is a vascular abnormality, it is typically a fine mosaic or a fine punctation. The tiles are small, homogenous, and intercapillary distances between vascular channels are normal (Figure 6–8c).

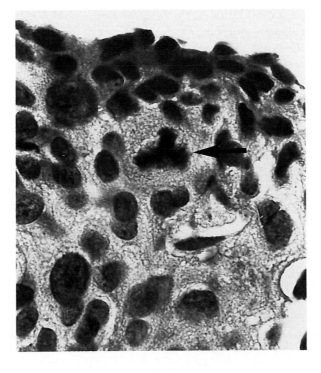

Figure 6–3. High power view of high grade CIN with an abnormal tripolar mitotic form *(arrow)*.

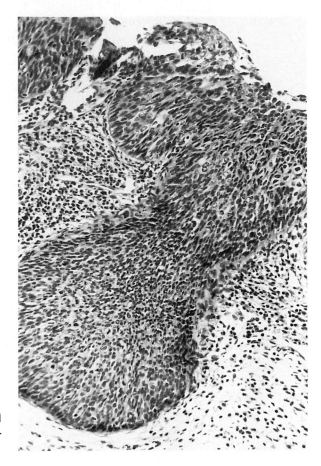

Figure 6-4. CIN III involving full thickness of the mucosa and endocervical invagination.

Cervical Intraepithelial Neoplasia II

In CIN II the cellular abnormality involves the lower two thirds of the epithelium, with some degree of maturation at the surface (Figure 6-9). Cytologically, the cells of CIN II have only modest amounts of cytoplasm, which tends to be more dense and basophilic than that of normal cells or the cells of CIN I (Figure 6-10). Nuclei are larger than in CIN I; they may be irregular in shape and will be obviously hyperchromatic, with aberrations of chromatin pattern.

Colposcopically, the lesions are distinctive (Figure 6-11). The aceto-whiteness appears rather quickly, lasts for several minutes, and fades slowly. The surface is usually flat, but the margin is sharp and distinct. It is not unusual for the lesion to have either a punctate or mosaic appearance. Although the blocks in mosaic areas may vary in size and shape, there is not a great deal of widening of the vascular channels or an increase in the intercapillary distances. The punctate vessels tend to be rather fine, with no increase in the intercapillary distances between the punctate vessels.

Cervical Intraepithelial Neoplasia III

In CIN III, abnormal cells occupy most or all of the epithelial thickness (Figure 6-12). Cytologically, the cells in CIN III have large nuclei with a markedly increased nuclear:cytoplasmic ratio (Figure 6-13). Hyperchromasia and chromatin aberrations are prominent, and the cytoplasm is reduced to a thin rim of densely staining material. These changes are typical of the so-called small cell, or nonkeratinizing type, of dysplasia. In keratinizing dysplasia, cytoplasm remains relatively more copious and tends to be orange-yellow; however, the nuclear aberrations are identical to those of the small cell nonkeratinizing type (Figure 6-14).

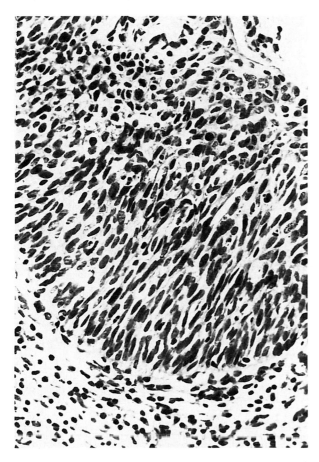

Figure 6-5. High power view of CIN III. Hyperchromatic basaloid cells occupy the entire thickness without surface maturation.

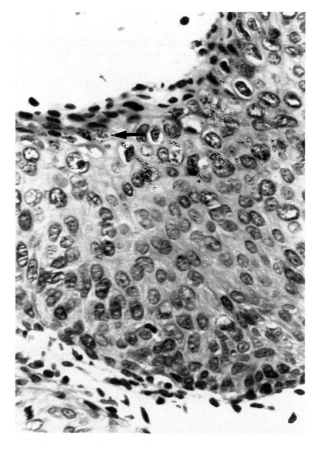

Figure 6-6. High grade dysplasia with keratinization. Note the keratohyaline granules (*arrow*).

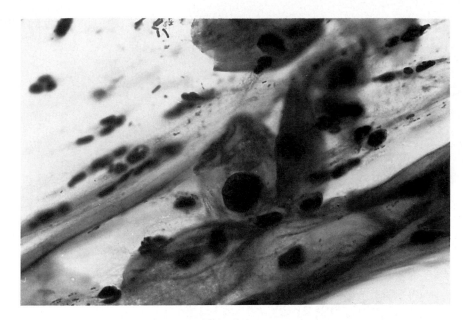

Figure 6-7. Cytosmear with CIN I. Note the cell in the center of the field with the enlarged and hyperchromatic nucleus; however, the nuclear:cytoplasmic ratio is not significantly altered.

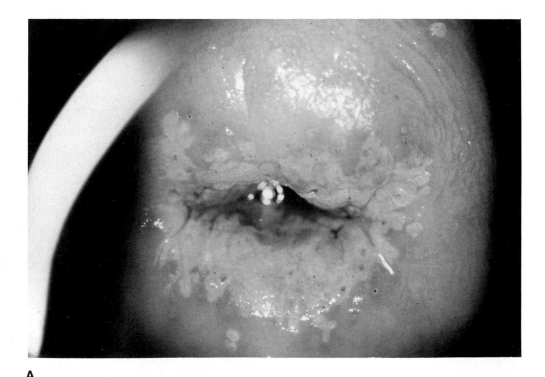

A

Figure 6-8. A. Colpophotograph after acetic acid. There is a grade I aceto-white change that is flat and has feathery borders. Biopsy revealed CIN I with koilocytosis. (*Figure continues.*)

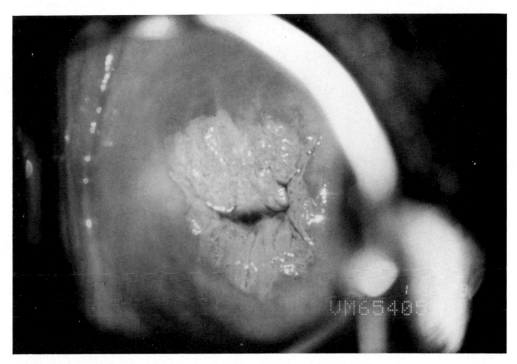

B

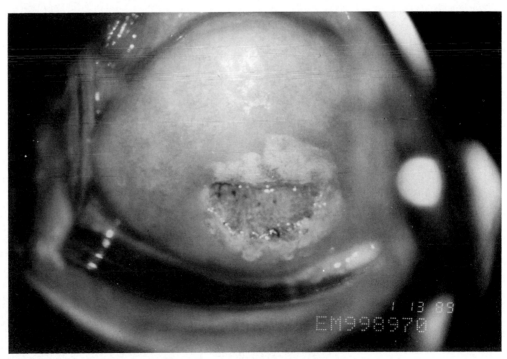

C

Figure 6–8 (continued).   B. Cervix after the application of acetic acid. There is opacity to a grade I white change at the periphery of the columnar epithelium at 10 to 11 and 6 o'clock. The margins of the lesion are not very distinct. Biopsy revealed CIN I. **C.** Grade I atypical transformation zone with a flat, aceto-white change at 5 to 10 and 4 o'clock. At 12 to 1 o'clock, a very fine punctate process is present. Biopsy of this area revealed CIN Grade I.

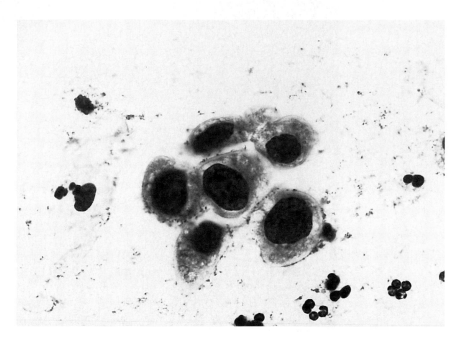

Figure 6-9. Biopsy specimen of CIN II. Abnormal cells extend through two thirds of mucosal thickness.

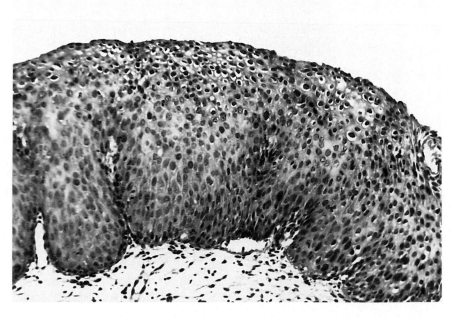

Figure 6-10. CIN II in cytologic smear. In contrast to CIN I, there is significantly less cytoplasm with a higher nuclear:cytoplasmic ratio.

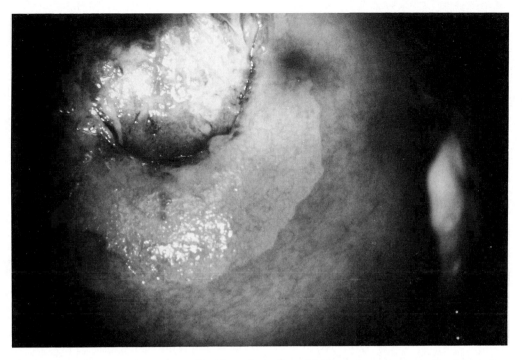

Figure 6-11. Cervix after the application of acetic acid. There is a large atypical transformation zone. On the posterior cervical lip there is a lesion with a sharp border and grade II mosaic change. At 1 o'clock on the anterior lip there is a grade II to III aceto-white change with some punctation. Biopsy revealed CIN II.

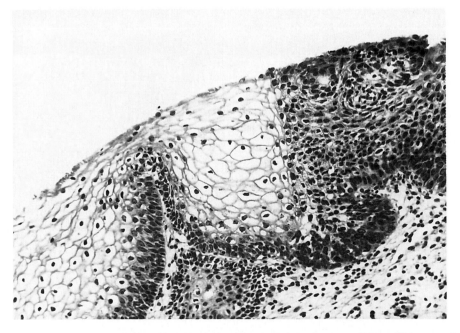

Figure 6-12. CIN, grade III, with full thickness cellular abnormalities. This specimen demonstrates the sharp demarcation of CIN with normal squamous mucosa of the portio.

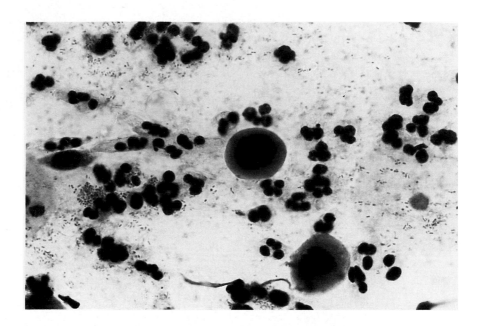

Figure 6-13. Cytologic specimen demonstrating CIN III (keratinizing type). Although the nucleus is smaller than that of cells with CIN I, the nuclear:cytoplasmic ratio is markedly altered.

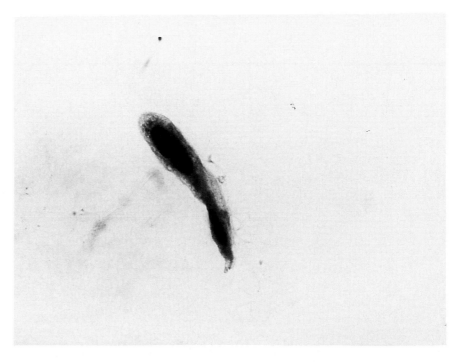

Figure 6-14. Cytosmear of keratinizing dysplasia. Note the abnormal cell shape, which is spindled, and the pyknotic nucleus.

Colposcopically, the lesions of CIN III are very dramatic (Figure 6–15a, Figure 6–15b, Color Plate 13). The surfaces are usually raised and undulating, with very sharp margins that may be "rolled" and also raised. The degree of whiteness is extreme, and various observers use terms such as "oyster white" or "ivory white" to describe the change. After the application of acetic acid, the lesions come up very rapidly, remain a long time, and fade slowly. Cervical interepithelial neoplasia III lesions usually contain some degree of vascular aberration in the form of punctation, mosaic, and possibly, atypical blood vessels. The tiles of the mosaic typically are rather pleomorphic and often contain a central punctate vessel. Vascular channels are wide, with a marked increase in intercapillary distances. The punctation usually is described as "coarse" in that each vessel seems to protrude above the surface of the lesion. If atypical vessels are identified, microinvasion or invasive disease should be considered (*see* Chapter 7) (Figure 6–16).

LOCATION AND NATURAL HISTORY OF CERVICAL INTRAEPITHIAL NEOPLASIA

The majority of CIN lesions develop in islands of metaplastic tissue within the transformation zone (TZ). A minority of lesions appear to arise on the portio of the cervix, lateral to the "last gland." A single or multiple foci of immature squamous metaplasia may undergo neoplastic transformation to CIN within the TZ. Multiple foci may enlarge, then coalesce, in some cases.

The distal margin of most CIN lesions is at the original squamocolumnar junction and presents a sharp demarcation from the adjacent normal exocervical mucosa. This sharp demarcation can be appreciated both histologically and colposcopically (Figure 6–17). Extention of lesions onto the portio does not occur unless invasive disease develops. Proximally, CIN lesions tend to involve the endocervical invaginations, as well as the surface, and to grow freely up the canal (Figure 6–18, Color Plate 14). The upward growth appears to be due to the "wedging out" of normal cells by the neoplastic element. In CIN lesions having a marked longitudinal extent, the most severe degree of dysplasia tends to be at the upper end of the lesion. This observation explains the importance of visualizing and sampling the upper end of all CIN lesions during colposcopy. Involvement of the endocervical invaginations should be noted on the pathology report in order to allow the clinician to tailor the depth of the ablative therapy appropriately.

DIFFERENTIAL DIAGNOSIS OF CERVICAL INTRAEPITHELIAL NEOPLASIA

Although the pathologist can make the diagnosis of CIN, he or she cannot predict the biologic behavior of true CIN in a particular patient by examining a biopsy specimen. The weight of evidence suggests that the majority of CIN from grade I through grade III, have the potential to persist or to progress to a higher grade of abnormality or to invasive carcinoma if no clinical intervention occurs. This sequence is by no means inevitable. The time required for progression varies greatly among the patients at risk. Given these variables, the pathologist realistically can be expected only to render a morphologic interpretation; therapy by the clinician should be aimed at eradication of the CIN regardless of its degree and should be based on factors such as the location and size of the lesion and the presence or absence of an associated invasive component.

Other diagnostic difficulties relate to the fact that a variety of non-neoplastic cervical lesions can mimic some aspects of CIN in biopsy specimens. Atrophy exhibits a lack of maturation in that the squamous epithelium consists primarily of basal and parabasal cells with relatively large nuclei and modest amounts of cytoplasm (*see* Figure 3–10). Mitotic activity, however, is minimal, and there is no significant nuclear atypia. Infectious or inflammatory processes or both, such as those caused by trichomonas

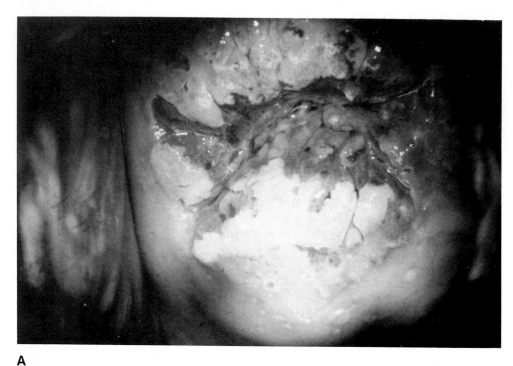

A

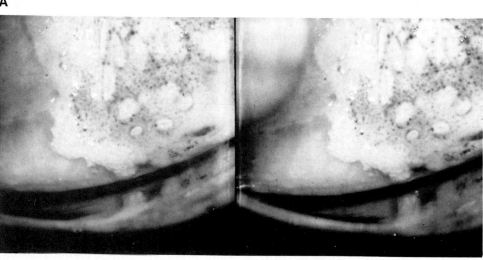

B

Figure 6–15. A. Posterior lip of the cervix after acetic acid. There is a sharply delineated, raised, grade III aceto-white lesion. Biopsy revealed CIN III. **B.** Posterior lip of cervix after acetic acid. The atypical transformation zone has a raised, grade III aceto-white lesion with sharp distinct border. Coarse punctation with increased intercapillary distances is very evident. This type of lesion could represent any degree of abnormality from CIN III to early invasive carcinoma.

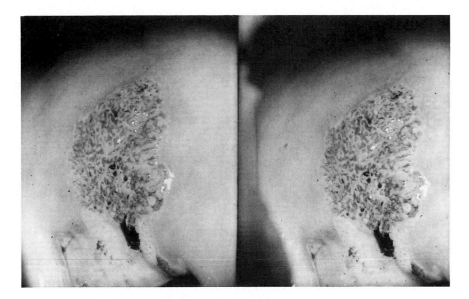

Figure 6-16. Cervix with a cluster of atypical blood vessels. Biopsy revealed microinvasive squamous cell carcinoma.

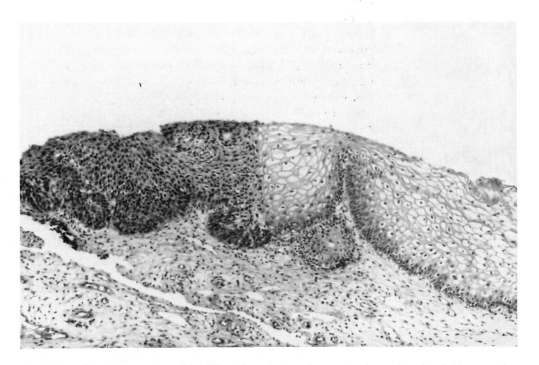

Figure 6-17. Biopsy of a CIN III lesion. Note the very sharp border between the neoplastic tissue and the normal epithelium.

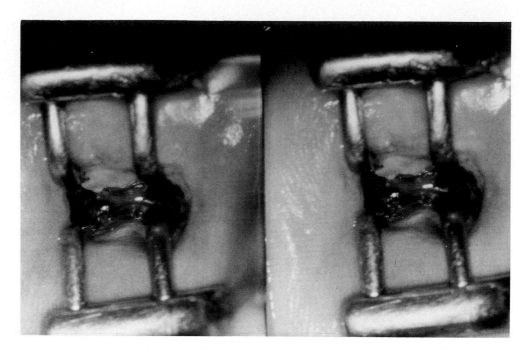

Figure 6-18. Colpophotograph of endocervical canal being visualized with an endocervical speculum. A lesion can be seen going up the canal for 1.5 cm. The upper edge of the lesion can be seen.

or trauma, are associated with intraepithelial inflammation, cell destruction, and an increased cell replication rate. The morphologic expression of these events is an epithelium formed by immature cells with enlarged nuclei and an increased mitotic index. On careful inspection, however, chromatin aberrations and abnormal mitotic figures (major hallmarks of true CIN) are not identified.

Immature squamous metaplasia of endocervical epithelium in the TZ is a major source of morphologic confusion in the differential diagnosis of CIN. Developing and maturing metaplastic epithelium exhibits mitotic activity and cells with increased nuclear:cytoplasmic ratios throughout much or all of its thickness (Figure 6-19). Cytoplasmic maturation is delayed, even in advanced metaplasia; the epithelium, therefore, is poorly glycogenated. Thus, it is easy to understand how metaplasia can mimic CIN, particularly in less than optimal tissue preparations (*see* Figure 4-16). As with the evaluation of inflammatory lesions, the absence of both nuclear aberrations and abnormal mitotic figures signifies a non-neoplastic process.

In the differential diagnosis of CIN, the current area of most intensive investigation is the distinction between banal condylomas and true neoplasia (*see* Chapter 10).

SCREENING AND DIAGNOSIS OF CERVICAL INTRAEPITHELIAL NEOPLASIA

Several techniques, which may be used singly or in combination, are available for the detection and diagnosis of cervical neoplasia. They are:

1. Cytology.
2. Colposcopy.
3. Cervicography.

Each technique has certain limitations that must be recognized in order to use it most effectively.

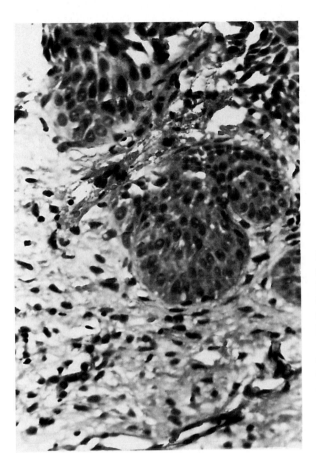

Figure 6-19. Histologic section of immature squamous metaplasia. The nodules of immature cells in the stroma represent cervical invaginations replaced by squamous epithelium. The immaturity of the cells is documented by their dense cytoplasm, which lacks glycogen, and by the relatively bland nuclei. Immature metaplastic cells are also present at the top of the photograph, on the surface of the biopsy.

Cytology

Exfoliative cytology, in use for over 40 years, is generally agreed to be the best available screening method for detecting cervical neoplasia. Although cervical cytology is economical and, theoretically, is easily performed, it has proven to have significant limitations in practice. These limitations will be discussed in Chapter 13.

Colposcopy

Colposcopy is the ideal means of evaluating patients with an abnormal cytosmear. Although cytology is highly accurate in predicting the presence of cervical neoplasia, it cannot determine its extent or location. By using colposcopy, however, the clinician can easily determine the location and extent of the neoplastic lesion, eliminating the need for diagnostic conization in over 90% of cases. It must be emphasized that colposcopy as it is performed in South America and in some parts of Europe is not recommended as a screening technique. Colposcopy requires constant practice in order for the colposcopist to achieve and retain a high level of accuracy. Colposcopy is also time consuming, taking 20 to 30 minutes to examine a patient adequately. The logistics and costs, therefore, prevent this method from being used as a screening tool. Cytology and cervicography are the screening methods of choice. The efficacy of colposcopic-directed

TABLE 6-1. DIAGNOSIS OF CERVICAL CANCER: ACCURACY OF CYTOLOGY AND COLPOSCOPY

Author	Cytologic Accuracy (%)	Colposcopic Accuracy (%)	Joint Accuracy (%)
Limburg (1958)	89	97	99
Navratil (1964)	87	79	99
Coppleson (1967)	93	92	98
Cope (1969)	90	95	95
Dexeus (1972)	91	94	99

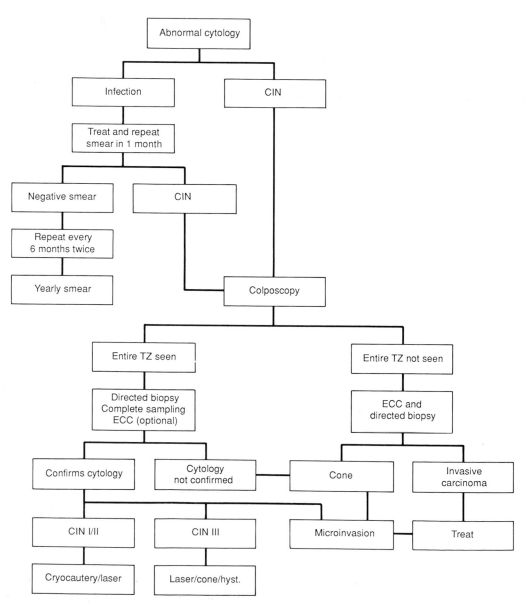

Figure 6-20. Allogram for investigating the atypical cytosmear.

biopsies can be seen on Table 6–1. Using cytology for screening and colposcopy for directing the biopsy, a joint accuracy of approximately 95% to 99% can be achieved.

Although colposcopy is extremely useful in evaluating the patient with an abnormal smear, an excisional conization must be performed if any of the conditions listed below pertain to the patient.

1. The entire cervical lesion is not visualized at colposcopy.
2. A persistently abnormal smear is obtained, with no colposcopic abnormality of the cervix, vagina, or vulva.
3. A colposcopic-directed biopsy reveals microinvasion.
4. A colposcopic biopsy demonstrates a two-grade difference of CIN from that detected by cytology.
5. An endocervical curettage (ECC) reveals CIN II or III.
6. CIN II or III occurs in patients unreliable for follow-up.
7. Large CIN II or III lesions present, for which laser therapy is not available.
8. Persistent CIN II or III are found after cryo or laser treatment.

Cervicography

A new modality, cervicography, has been developed for screening the cervix. This will be discussed in Chapter 14.

TREATMENT OF CERVICAL INTRAEPITHELIAL NEOPLASIA

The treatment of CIN may be divided into those cases that are amenable to ablative therapy and those that meet the criteria noted in the preceding list and require an excisional conization. If the latter is not indicated, a variety of methodologies are available such as laser vaporization, cryotherapy, Sem's cold coagulation, electrodiathermy, and electrocoagulation. All of these modalities may be utilized successfully in treating CIN.

Figure 6–20 is an allogram suggesting the method for following an abnormal cytosmear.

Chapter 7

Colposcopy of Microinvasive and Invasive Cancer of the Cervix

MICROINVASIVE SQUAMOUS CELL CARCINOMA

Microinvasive carcinoma (MIC), represents preclinical invasive disease (stage IA). It represents the earliest phase of invasive squamous cell carcinoma, in which there is essentially no risk of metastatic disease. The diagnosis implies rigorous examination of a cone biopsy specimen to exclude more extensive invasion.

Histology

Histologically, MIC consists of tongues or nests of neoplastic cells extending into the stroma from the epithelium of either the cervical surface or invaginations. The invading groups of cells are usually irregular in shape (unlike the smooth contour of cervical intraepithelial neoplasia [CIN] confined to invaginations) and are often accompanied by a lymphocytic infiltrate. In addition, the invasive cells are often more keratinized than those of the overlying CIN (Figure 7-1).

Cytology

The cytologic features of microinvasive squamous carcinoma are intermediate between those of carcinoma in situ and frankly malignant disease. The cells, which may be shed within synctia or singly, have hyperchromatic nuclei with an irregular nuclear membrane and a high nuclear:cytoplasmic ratio. The chromatin pattern is irregular and finely granular, in contrast to the regular, coarsely granular chromatin pattern of carcinoma in situ. Micronucleoli and a tumor diathesis (fresh and old blood, granular proteinaceous background, inflammatory cells, and necrotic debris) may also be seen (Figure 7-2a, 7-2b).

Colposcopy

The colposcopic appearance of MIC is similar in many ways to that of invasive carcinoma. The unexpected recognition of clusters of atypical blood vessels in an area of high-grade CIN should alert the colposcopist to the possibility that the epithelial basement membrane has been breached by neoplastic cells (Figure 7-3, Color Plate 15). These atypical vessels may occur anywhere within the CIN lesion but often are located at its

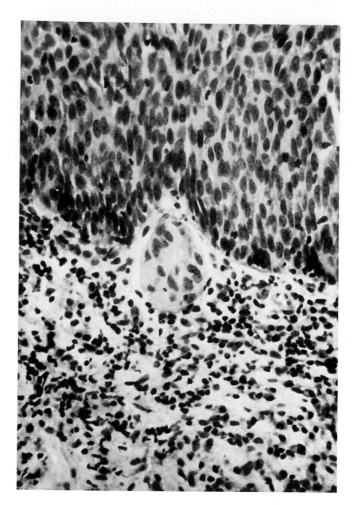

Figure 7-1. Microinvasive cervical carcinoma. A nodule of keratinized invasive cells is in the stroma beneath a high grade CIN lesion.

periphery. The vessels tend to be clumped and irregular in size and shape. Although increasing intercapillary distances are the hallmarks of increasing severity of intraepithelial neoplasia, the intercapillary distances are often less than normal in MIC because of the neovascularization that is characteristic of early invasive disease. The vessels, which are admixed with tufted, punctate capillaries, tend to be very friable, so that as nontraumatic a procedure as washing the cervix with acetic acid may produce bleeding and subepithelial distortion. In addition to atypical blood vessels, the foci of MIC may have an abnormal color and an uneven, raised surface contour.

Diagnosis

The major controversy in defining MIC is determining the maximum allowable depth of invasion that carries no significant risk of metastatic disease and for which, therefore, less than radical surgery is indicated. Unfortunately, no precise and universally accepted definition of MIC exists: the permitted depth of invasion into the stroma (as measured from the base of the mucosa) has varied from as little as 1.0 mm, to 3.0 mm (SGO definition) or 5.0 mm (new FIGO classification). Some workers will exclude a case if capillary-lymphatic space invasion is identified even if stromal invasion is minimal, whereas others will exclude cases showing "confluent tumor growth" (an ill-defined concept) or a large tumor volume (difficult to evaluate unless numerous, subserial sections are obtained).

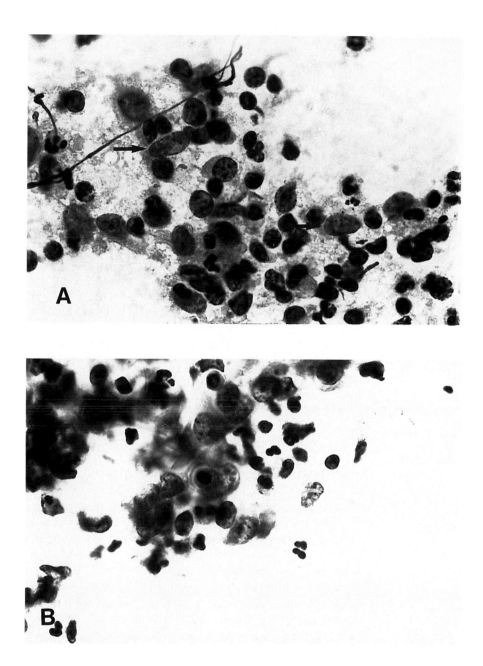

Figure 7-2.   A. Cytology of microinvasive squamous cell carcinoma. The arrows mark single malignant cells surrounded by acute and chronic inflammatory cells. The chromatin pattern is irregular and finely granular, with micronucleoli, and there is a background of inflammatory cells, necrotic debris, fibrin, and old and fresh red blood cells, all of which constitute a tumor diathesis. **B.** Microinvasive squamous cell carcinoma with loosely cohesive three-dimensional aggregrate of cells called a syncytium. The nuclei are markedly irregular, with micronucleoli.

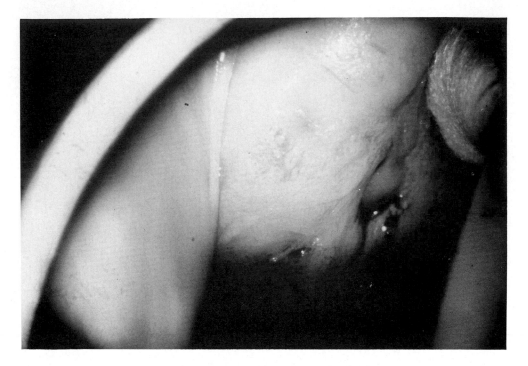

Figure 7-3. Cervix after application of acetic acid. A cluster of atypical blood vessels stands out in a field of aceto-white epithelium at 9 o'clock.

Management

Despite the current lack of a uniform definition of MIC, certain guidelines for management may be proposed. If stromal invasion is 1.0 mm or less and no capillary-lymphatic space invasion is identified, then the risk of nodal metastases is zero. Similarly, nodal metastases are absent in virtually all patients with invasion up to 3.0 mm and negative capillary-lymphatic spaces (SGO definition). If stromal invasion ranges between 3.1 and 5.0 mm, however, nodal metastases has been noted in 2% to 14% of patients in various series. Thus, conservative management for MIC should be considered (1) only after careful examination of a cone biopsy specimen by a pathologist familiar with the nuances of this entity; and (2) if stromal invasion is 3.0 mm or less in depth, as measured from the base of the mucosa. Vascular space invasion, if present, should be noted, although it is not clear that it is a factor of independent significance in predicting metastatic disease.

In addition, some workers have advocated inclusion of the colposcopic appearance among the factors determining whether radical or conservative therapy is to be employed. If the colposcopic appearance is primarily that of CIN III with a small area of atypical blood vessels, a conservative approach may be considered. On the other hand, if the lesion fits the colposcopic criteria for the category termed "invasion cannot be ruled out," then a conservative method of treatment would perhaps be hazardous. Lesions that are worrisome tend to have large numbers of atypical blood vessels, very uneven surfaces, a grade III-type coloration, and raised, sharp, curled borders (*see* Chapters 5, 6, and Figure 6-15b). Lesions of this type should be viewed with the suspicion that true invasive disease is present somewhere within them, even if histologic examination of cone biopsy specimens defines features compatible only with microinvasion.

INVASIVE SQUAMOUS CELL CARCINOMA

Histology

Frankly invasive cervical squamous cell carcinoma exhibits a wide spectrum of histologic appearances encompassing well- to poorly-differentiated tumors and numerous subtypes, such as glassy cell carcinoma. With the exception, however, of the small cell variant, which is actually of neuroendocrine origin, histologic grading is of less prognostic significance than the depth of invasion, the presence of vascular space involvement, and direct extension to adjacent organs. Invasive squamous cell carcinomas are often at least focally eroded or ulcerated at their surfaces due to ischemic necrosis, with a prominent secondary inflammatory response. The tumors also often elicit a desmoplastic stromal response (Figure 7–4).

Cytology

Invasive carcinoma presents a cytologic picture of a pronounced tumor diathesis containing many single malignant cells whose nuclei have an irregular, coarsely granular chromatin pattern and macronucleoli. Such smears tend to be very hypercellular. In keratinizing carcinomas, many cells with abnormal shapes are identified. They may be elongated and spindle-shaped with central nuclei (strap cells) or elongated with an eccentrically located nucleus (tadpole cells). Their cytoplasm is dense and orangophilic, and the nuclear chromatin tends to be dense and smudged. The non-keratinizing type of squamous carcinoma sheds single cells with amphophilic cytoplasm. Macronucleoli are common in this type of carcinoma, and chromatin clumping may be so pronounced as to leave clear areas ("holes") in the nucleus. The small cell variant of squamous carcinoma also sheds single cells that are small and characterized by nuclei with dense, hyperchromatic, coarsely granular chromatin surrounded by a thin rim of cytoplasm (Figure 7–5).

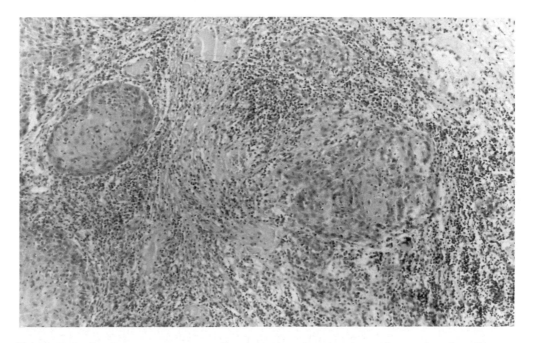

Figure 7–4. Invasive squamous cell carcinoma showing irregular nests of malignant cells in the stroma.

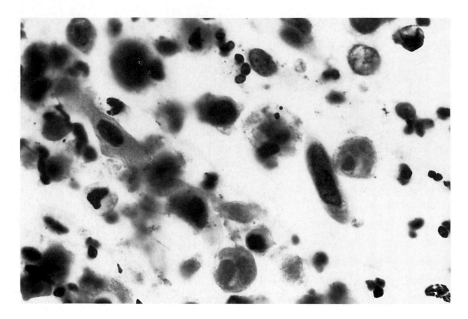

Figure 7-5. Cytosmear compatible with invasive squamous cell carcinoma. There is a background of necrotic debris (tumor diathesis), and the neoplastic cellular nuclei are hyperchromatic and vary in shape. Note the elongated, cigar-shaped nucleus in the right half of the photograph.

Colposcopy

The colposcopic appearance of invasive squamous cell carcinoma reflects the underlying histopathology. Irrespective of the extent of disease, its hallmark is the presense of atypical blood vessels. These vessels tend to be much more numerous and extensive than those characteristic of microinvasive disease; however, a colposcopic distinction between these two conditions cannot be made. Loss of mucosal surface integrity with progression of invasive disease is an obvious finding colposcopically, and one which, along with the presence of atypical vessels, suggests invasion. The atypical vessels are usually very bizarre, and all types of strange shapes (spaghetti, commas, thick–thin–thick, etc) may occur. The vessels are very friable and bleed on touch (Figure 7-6, Color Plate 15, Color Plate 16). Because of the necrosis that accompanies frank invasion, the lesion will have a yellowish hue (Color Plate 17). Obvious exophytic lesions will be ulcerated and necrotic; colposcopy is not necessary to make the diagnosis. The student who wishes to study abnormal blood vessels, however, would do well to look at these lesions colposcopically. At the edge and in the non-necrotic areas of the carcinoma, the grossly abnormal vessels will be quite apparent.

ADENOCARCINOMA OF THE ENDOCERVIX

Adenocarcinoma of the endocervix has increased in relative frequency in the past two decades and now accounts for up to 18% of all primary exo- and endocervical cancers. In addition, more cases (15% to 35%) are occurring in women 35 years or younger. Both in situ and invasive endocervical adenocarcinoma have been documented to contain human papilloma virus (HPV) DNA, particularly for genotypes 18, and up to 50% of women with endocervical cancers will also have CIN.

The primary clinical sign of endocervical adenocarcinoma is vaginal bleeding, which is noted in 75% of women. Patients with endocervical adenocarcinoma have an increased risk of developing primary ovarian neoplasms, chiefly of the mullerian type, and

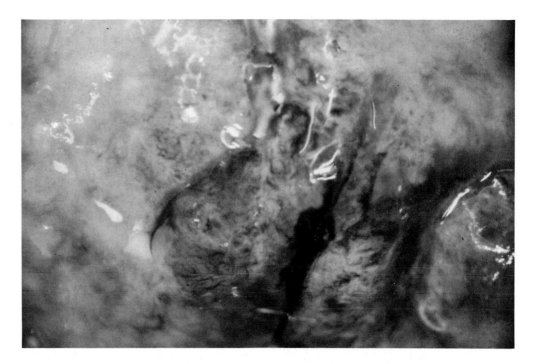

Figure 7-6.   Portion of cervix with invasive squamous cell carcinoma. Numerous atypical blood vessels are present and are irregular in shape, **parallel to the surface**, nondividing, and friable.

endocervical cancers may also be more frequent in women with the Peutz-Jeghers syndrome. There is no convincing evidence, however, of associations with oral contraceptive use, microglandular hyperplasia, or exposure to diethylstilbestrol (DES) in utero.

Histology

Histologically, endocervical adenocarcinomas are variable in appearance, but the majority recapitulate mullerian types (endometrioid, clear cell, endocervical, mucinous, and papillary). Minimal deviation variants (adenoma malignum) may look deceptively benign under the microscope except for their extension deep into the endocervical stroma (Figure 7-7). The endocervical neoplasms spread in a manner similar to that of cervical squamous cell carcinoma, but a larger percentage of the endocervical tumors are clinically advanced at the time of detection.

Cytology

Cytologically, the cells that exfoliate from endocervical adenocarcinoma in situ present as loosely or more tightly cohesive sheets of cells in a palisade pattern, often with pseudostratified nuclei and rosette formation. The cells are columnar with an enlarged, oval, hyperchromatic nucleus with granular chromatin and, sometimes, granular nucleoli. The cytoplasm may be finely vacuolated or granular. Synctia, papillary groupings, small cells in crowded sheets, single cells, a tumor diathesis, and macronucleoli all suggest invasion. The minimal deviation form of endocervical adenocarcinoma is a special problem; cells are generally bland or only minimally atypical (Figure 7-8).

Colposcopy

Colposcopically, the appearances of adenocarcinoma involving the endocervix are not specific or characteristic; they are the findings usually associated with invasive cancer (Color Plate 16, Color Plate 18). Some investigators have tried to correlate the width

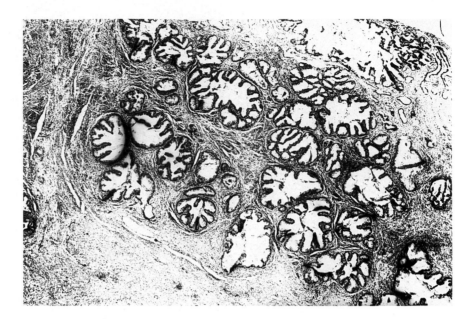

Figure 7–7. Endocervical adenocarcinoma with well-differentiated glands extending deep into the stroma.

of the atypical vessels with the possibility of an adenocarcinoma; namely, that in the latter, the vessels seem to be wider than in invasive squamous cell carcinoma. The tumors are most often polypoid or ulcerated masses, but in approximately 20% of women no lesion is visible either because the neoplasm is too small, is too high up in the canal, or is hidden within an endocervical cleft.

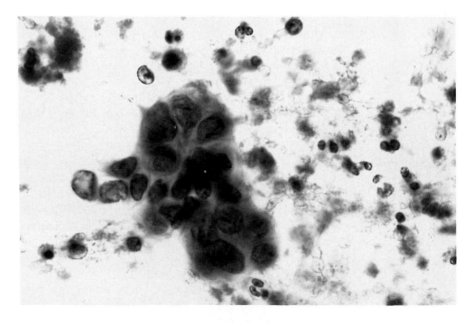

Figure 7–8. Cytology of endocervical adenocarcinoma. Note the glandular cluster of atypical cells with enlarged and irregular nuclei in a background of a tumor diathesis.

Diagnosis

In terms of diagnosis, cytosmears have been reported as positive in 45% to 95% of patients. False-negatives may be related to the small size of some tumors, their inaccessible location, lack of experience in recognizing these often well-differentiated tumors on the part of the cytologist, or inadequate sampling. The highest diagnostic yield is a sample obtained by endocervical aspiration or by use of the cytobrush in the canal. Endocervical and endometrial curettage also aid in the correct diagnosis. The definitive diagnosis of endocervical carcinoma requires histologic examination of either biopsies or a cervical cone specimen. In situ adenocarcinoma is a diagnosis of exclusion, based on careful examination of a cone biopsy specimen.

The 5-year survival rate is in the range of 45% to 55%; recurrences are noted in about 25% of women. Prognosis is not significantly related to the histologic type of the tumor but rather to the degree of tumor differentiation and to the clinical stage of the disease at the time of diagnosis.

Chapter 8 | Colposcopy of the Vagina

INDICATIONS AND TECHNIQUES

Colposcopy of the vagina is indicated:

1. To investigate the source of an abnormal cytologic smear following hysterectomy.
2. To evaluate the patient with an abnormal cytosmear but a normal cervix.
3. To evaluate patients with vulvar or cervical squamous intraepithelial neoplasia who are at risk for multifocal genital tract lesions.
4. To evaluate patients with human papilloma virus (HPV) infection.
5. To delineate further abnormal gross findings noted on pelvic examination.
6. To detect and monitor abnormalities in women who have been exposed in utero to diethylstilbestrol (DES).

Although the colposcopic lesions observed in the vagina are basically the same as those observed on the cervix (ie, aceto-white epithelium, mosaic structure, punctation, leukoplakia, and atypical blood vessels), their microscopic correlates differ somewhat from those of the cervix. The connective tissue of the vagina is looser and more abundant than that of the cervix, and the vasculature of the vagina is somewhat increased (Figure 8–1). Colposcopically, the normal vagina epithelium has a pink, smooth appearance with numerous rugae (Figure 8–2, *see* Color Plate 1). At higher magnification, the terminal capillary network, similar to that of the cervix, can be seen. In addition, except in the DES exposed female, there is no interface between the columnar and the stratified squamous epithelium and, therefore, no transformation zone (TZ) (*see* Figure 8–1, Figure 8–2). The appearances of vaginial lesions colposcopically tend to be exophytic, producing large papillomatous projections with dilated vascular cores. The colposcopic grade of a lesion in the vagina generally appears to be somewhat greater than that in the cervix for a particular histopathologic degree of intraepithelial neoplasia.

The colposcopic examination of the vagina is tedious and requires not only the usual application of acetic acid, but also the manipulation of all the folds and rugae. A hook or mirror may be necessary to investigate the angles of the vagina (Figure 8–3, Figure 8–4). Unlike other areas of the lower genital tract, use of Lugol's iodine solution is always necessary in colposcopy of the vagina (Figure 8–5, Color Plate 19).

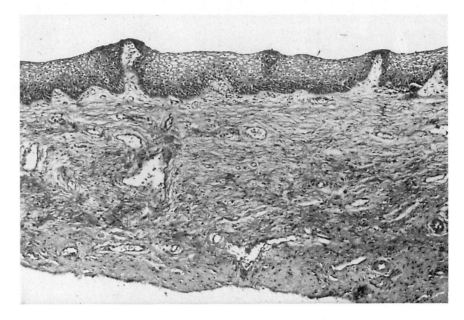

Figure 8-1. Normal vagina. The squamous mucosa is multilayered, with maturation to horizontally oriented superficial cells. The cytoplasm is clear due to the accumulation of glycogen. The stroma has numerous blood vessels and is less dense than that of the cervix.

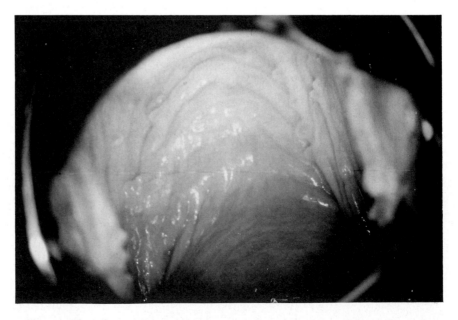

Figure 8-2. Colpophotograph of anterior fornix of normal vagina. The epithelium is unremarkable with numerous rugae and has a pink coloration (*see* Color Plate 1).

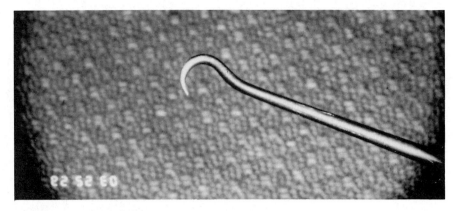

Figure 8-3. Burke hook for manipulating cervix, vagina, and vulva.

BIOPSY

As on the cervix, biopsy of the vagina can be done without the use of anesthesia. In order to minimize the discomfort of the patient, however, the instrument must be sharp (*see* Chapter 2). An Eppendorfer, Tischler, or Burke biopsy forceps will work well. Occasionally, one will have to "tent" the mucosa with a hook (Burke or Iris) to raise a ridge, which can then be readily biopsied. In general, the punch should cut across perpendicular to the vaginal ridges and folds to prevent slipping (Figure 8–6a, Figure 8–6b).

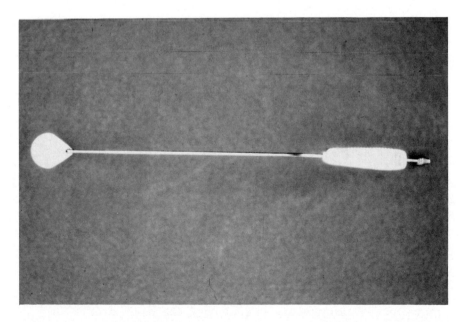

Figure 8-4. Polished stainless steel mirror used for visualizing out of the way areas in the vagina.

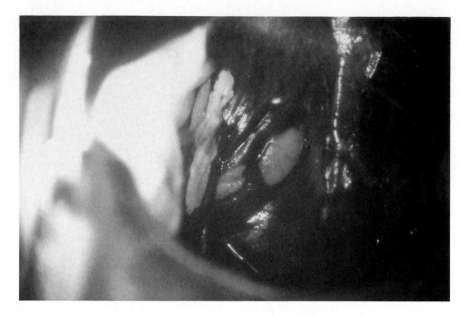

Figure 8-5. Vaginal mucosa after staining with 50% Lugol's iodine solution. Several raised areas of vaginal intraepithelial neoplasia grade III do not take the stain.

CONDITIONS IDENTIFIED THROUGH COLPOSCOPY

Some conditions commonly identified during colposcopy of the vagina are described in the following sections.

Leukoplakia

Leukoplakia of the vagina may develop in three clinical situations.

Use of Contraceptives. A common finding is thickening of the vaginal epithelium in association with prolonged use of the diaphragm as a means of contraception. The acidic nature of the jelly used to lubricate the diaphragm is believed to stimulate the vaginal epithelium, which becomes hypertrophied, thus producing thickened rugae with a somewhat opaque coloration. No abnormal vascular changes are noted, and the main histologic feature on biopsy is acanthosis. The layers of squamous cells are increased, but maturation is normal. Keratohyline granules develop in the superficial squamous cells. Although parakeratosis is uncommon, a layer of surface keratin of variable thickness is usually present (Figure 8-7, Figure 8-8).

Human Papilloma Viral Infection. A second common cause of vaginal mucosal thickening with a white papillary appearance is infection by viruses of the HPV group. Such condylomas may manifest in any of three ways. The first manifestation is the usual exophytic papillary lesion, characteristic of condylomas in any location. The epithelium is thickened and the vessels are usually not very clear; however, prominent vessels may, on occasion, impart a red color to some of the condylomas. Microscopically, the thickened (acanthotic) squamous epithelium is organized into very complex papillary folds whose cores are formed of connective tissues and blood vessels. In the typical exophytic condyloma accuminatum, the basal layer of the squamous epithelium is normal; however, the maturing squamous cells demonstrate the spectrum of HPV related changes: koilocytosis, variation in nuclear size and shape, some degree of nuclear chromatin aberration, multinucleation, or a combination of these. Mitosis may be numerous, but they

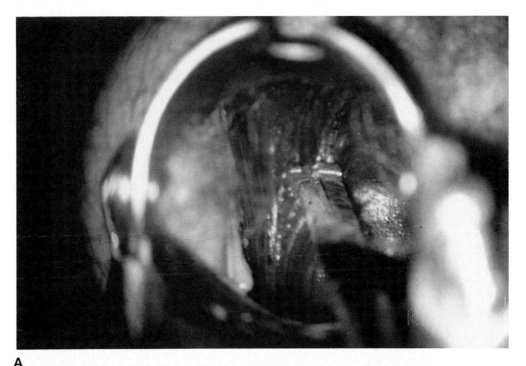

A

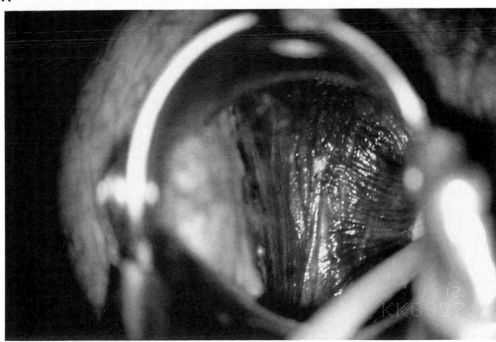

B

Figure 8-6. **A.** Biopsy of the vagina with the Burke punch. **B.** Biopsy site in the vagina.

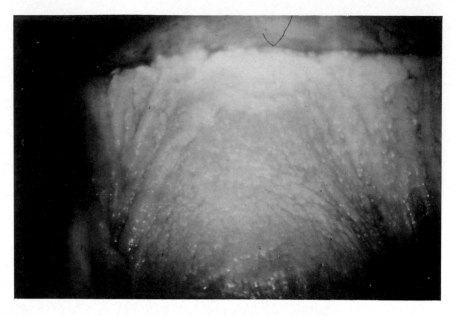

Figure 8-7.   Colpophotograph of the anterior fornix of the vagina of a patient with prolonged use of the diaphragm.

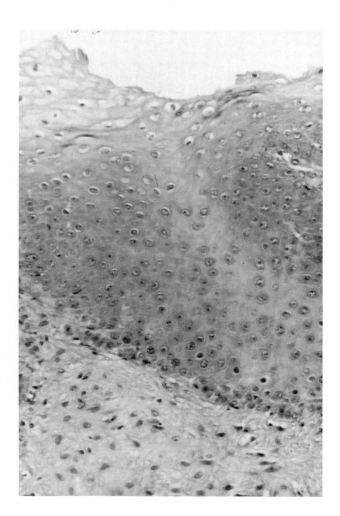

Figure 8-8. Pathology of the biopsy taken from the vagina in Figure 8-7. Note the acanthosis and dense cytoplasm of the squamous cells.

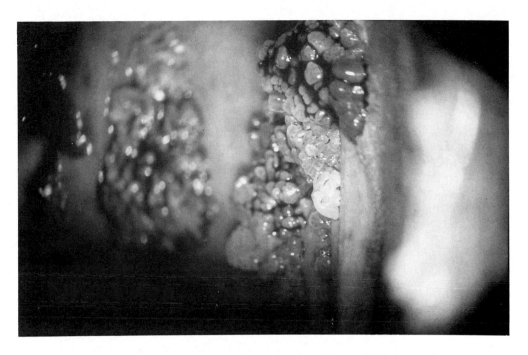

Figure 8-9.   Exophytic condyloma on the side wall of the vagina.

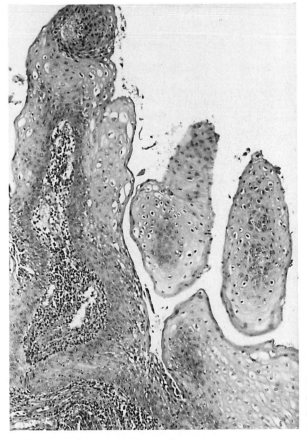

Figure 8-10.   Pathology of biopsy of Figure 8-9. Papillomatosis, acanthosis, koilocytosis, and parakeratosis are present.

have normal configurations. Parakeratosis may be noted, and keratin formation at the surface at the lesion may be prominent (hyperkeratosis) (Figure 8–9, Figure 8–10).

The second form of condylomas is of greater import, because it is often confused clinically with vaginal intraepithelial neoplasia. This type is the so-called "flat condyloma." It is slightly raised but lacks papillary projections. It is white, often multiple, ovoid, and usually occurs on the crest of the vaginal ridges. Flat condylomas may have a diffuse, even, punctate appearance, similar to that often seen with vaginal intraepithelial neoplasia. Examination of biopsy specimens, however, will show the characteristics of HPV infection. The histopathology is similar to that of the exophytic condyloma just described, with the exception that the architecture of the lesion is flat rather than papillary. Histologically, these are banal lesions; however, as discussed in the chapter on HPV infection (see Chapter 10) their biologic behavior cannot be predicted from their microscopic appearance (Figure 8–11, Figure 8–12).

The third variant of condyloma is the so-called "spiked lesion." Morphologically, this variant closely resembles the flat condyloma except for the presence of tiny surface projections (asperities) that extend into the surface epithelium and contain a capillary tip and a minimal amount of stroma. The cellular features of HPV infection described above often are only minimally evident in the spiked condyloma. Spiked lesions typically are tiny white plaques colposcopically; on occasion, they may be numerous and diffuse throughout the vagina, an appearance termed "condylomatosis vaginitis" (Figure 8–13, Figure 8–14). The cellular features of HPV infection in vaginal cytosmears are the same as those described in Chapter 10.

Use of Estrogen Creams. Leukoplakia of the vagina may also be seen in women exposed to large doses of estrogen, given either systemically or by means of topical application of estrogen creams. These raised white areas may be confused clinically with condylomas (Figure 8–15). Evaluation of biopsy material, however, demonstrates their true nature: normally maturing squamous epithelium without features of HPV infection, surmounted by a layer of keratin.

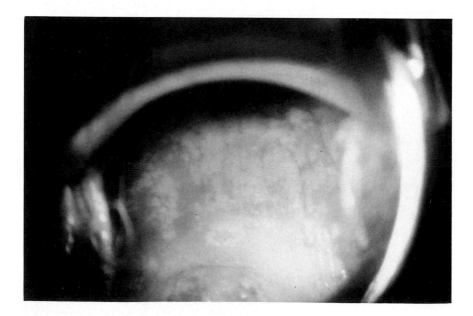

Figure 8–11. Posterior vaginal fornix after acetic acid. Numerous, flat aceto-white areas are present.

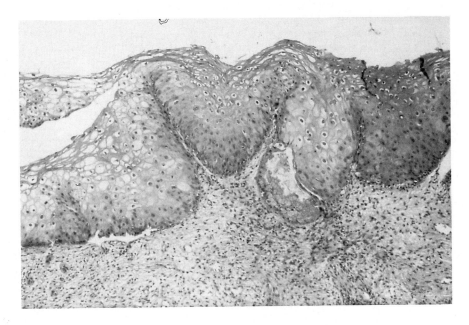

Figure 8-12. Biopsy of aceto-white areas of vagina in Figure 8-11 showing "flat" condyloma.

Other Papillomatous Lesions

Colposcopy may aid in elucidating the nature of polypoid lesions in the lateral vaginal fornices after hysterectomy for benign disease. The appearance of granulationlike tissue in these areas always raised the question of fallopian tube prolapse. Granulation tissue developing after total hysterectomy may seem to have many atypical vessels on initial evaluation; however, careful inspection of the vascular pattern will reveal tiny capillaries running in a smooth course, which is usually parallel to the surface. Frequently, two

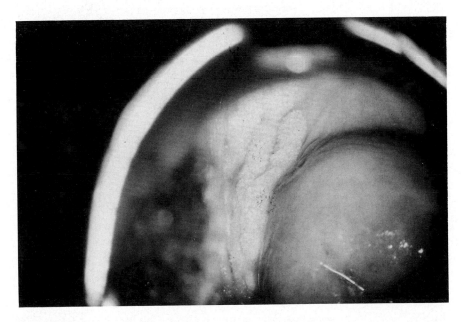

Figure 8-13. Vaginal fornix with condyloma containing "spiked" areas called "asperities."

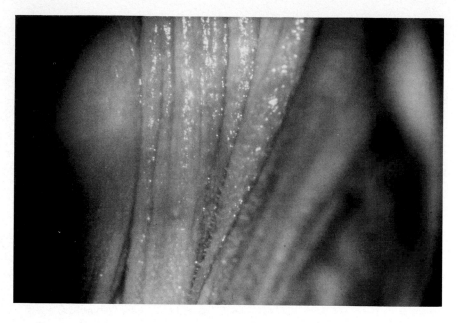

Figure 8-14. Side wall of vagina showing an early "spiked" condylomatous lesion with "asperities."

or more vessels will run parallel, then form a coil loop (Figure 8-16). Biopsy of these areas will delineate the true nature of the lesion. Granulation tissue will consist of proliferating small blood vessels and fibroblasts admixed with active and chronic inflammatory cells (Figure 8-17). Prolapsed fallopian tube, on the other hand, will be characterized by the presence of recognizable papillae, often associated with inflam-

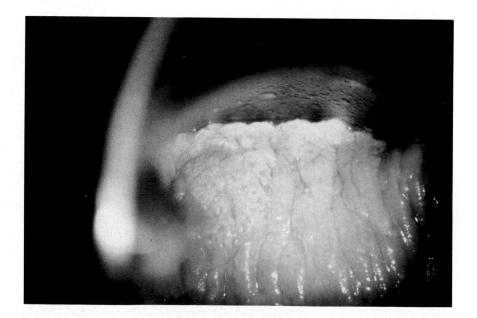

Figure 8-15. Anterior fornix of vagina of a patient on long-term estrogen therapy. Note the "cerebriform" character of the change, which resembles a lesion due to HPV infections.

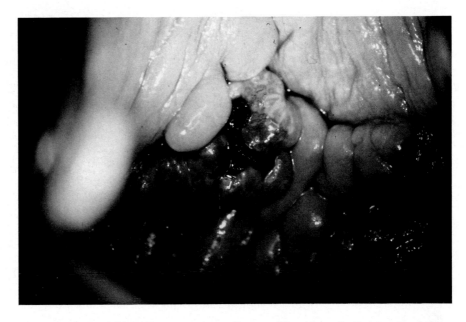

Figure 8-16. Granulation tissue surrounding a silk suture in the vault of the vagina after hysterectomy. Note the atypical blood vessels at the superior edge of the lesion.

mation or smooth muscle representing the tubal wall. At colposcopy, the prolapsed fallopian tube frequently will also demonstrate the mullerian nature of its epithelium. Prolapsed tubal plicae may have a somewhat papillary appearance after the application of 3% acetic acid, and their vessels tend to be very wide, with an arborization pattern characteristic of the normal vasculature of mullerian duct structures (Figure 8-18).

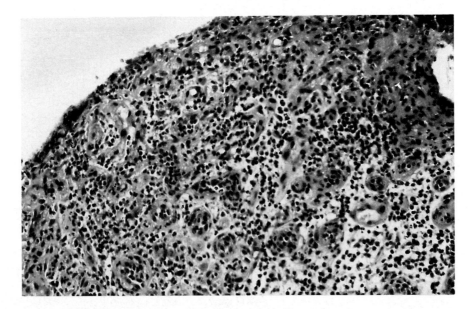

Figure 8-17. Granulation tissue in vagina with chronic inflammatory cells and capillary proliferation.

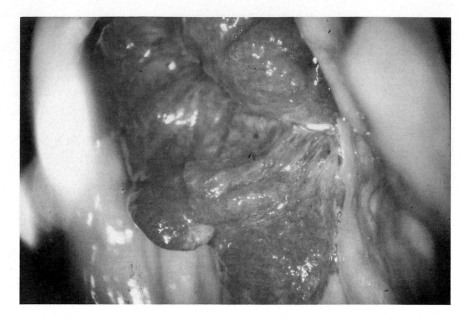

Figure 8-18. Vaginal vault after hysterectomy with a prolapsed Fallopian tube. Note the dividing vessels.

Atrophy of the Vagina

Colposcopic evaluation of the vagina may be instigated by receipt of the results of an abnormal cytosmear taken from atrophic vaginal mucosa in the postmenopausal woman. The abnormality may even suggest the presence of severe vaginal intraepithelial neoplasia (VaIN) or an invasive squamous tumor. The cytologic picture of vaginal atrophy is characterized by a maturation "shift to the left"; that is, by a preponderance of parabasal cells from the lower portion of the vaginal epithelium. Parabasal cells may undergo

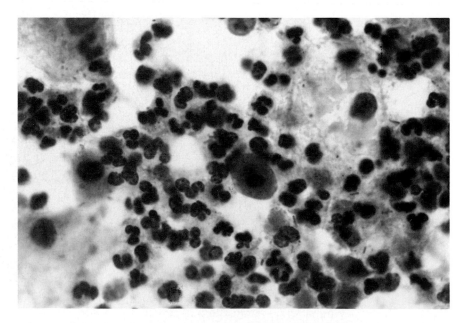

Figure 8-19. Cytology of an atrophic vagina. The atypical parabasal cell *(center of photo)* may be confused with true dysplasia.

degenerative changes and be confused with the necrotic surface cells associated with squamous carcinoma (Figure 8–19). Because this appearance may present a considerable diagnostic dilemma for the pathologist, an estrogen or proliferation test should be used when there is doubt about the correct interpretation. The patient is treated for 3 weeks with estrogen cream, and a repeat smear is taken. Under the influence of estrogen, atrophic parabasal cells will mature into intermediate and superficial squamous cells with clearing of background debris, whereas the cells of cancer remain atypical, with an associated tumor diathesis in the background.

At colposcopy, the vaginal vasculature of atrophy is readily recognized as being normal. The vessels are very friable (Figure 8–20). When acetic acid is applied, sub-epithelial hemorrhages occur frequently. No aceto-white lesions or other colposcopic abnormalities are seen. Examination of biopsy specimens from atrophic vaginal mucosa will document that the squamous epithelium is of diminished thickness and is composed predominantly of basal and parabasal cells. Because these are immature cells, their nuclear:cytoplasmic ratios are high throughout the thickness of the mucosa. On casual review, this immature epithelium may be confused with high-grade dysplasia because of the nuclear enlargement; however, careful inspection will reveal that nuclear chromatin aberrations are lacking and that mitoses, if present at all, have a normal configuration (Figure 8–21).

Vaginal atrophy developing over time, secondary to the use of radiation for the treatment of either invasive cervical carcinoma or endometrial carcinoma, is characterized by a thinned, friable epithelium associated with numerous atypical blood vessels. These subepithelial vessels have all the various shapes described for atypical vessels elsewhere (Figure 8–22).

Histologic examination of vaginal tissue with chronic radiation-induced changes shows an immature to frankly atrophic squamous epithelium and a variety of stromal changes, including enlarged fibroblasts with bizarre shaped and hyperchromatic nuclei, hyalinization of the walls (or complete obliteration of small blood vessels), and sclerosis of the stroma. In about one quarter of the patients who have had radiation for the treatment of cervical carcinoma, the squamous epithelium will contain abnormalities (nuclear enlargement, variable cytoplasmic maturation) resembling those of mild dysplasia.

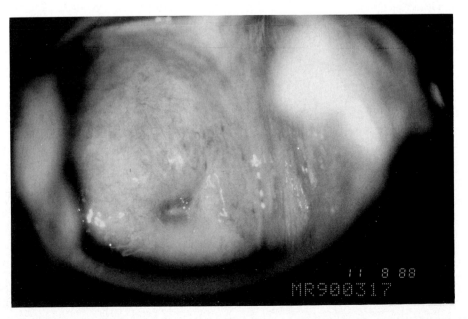

Figure 8–20.   Atrophic cervix and vagina prior to the application of acetic acid. Note the prominent vasculature.

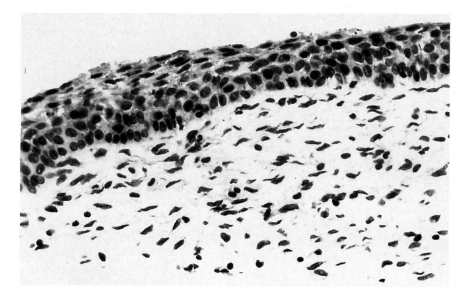

Figure 8-21. Atrophy of the vagina. The squamous mucosa is decreased in thickness and consists predominantly of parabasal and intermediate cells. There is a lack of maturation to superficial cells. The nuclei are relatively large but show no chromatin aberrations.

Radiation has long-term effects on the cytosmear. The changes related to radiation are similar to chemotherapy effect and to B-12/folate deficiency (Figure 8–23). There is nuclear enlargement, but the abundant cytoplasm maintains the normal nuclear:cytoplasmic ratio. Multinucleated cells are common with "two-tone," eosinophilic and cyanophilic cytoplasm. Cytoplasmic vacuoles, often with ingested leukocytes, are common. These changes do not indicate postradiation dysplasia; this term is reserved for a picture similar to dysplasia de novo in which an increased nuclear:cytoplasmic ratio, nuclear hyperchromasia, and a granular chromatin pattern are superimposed on

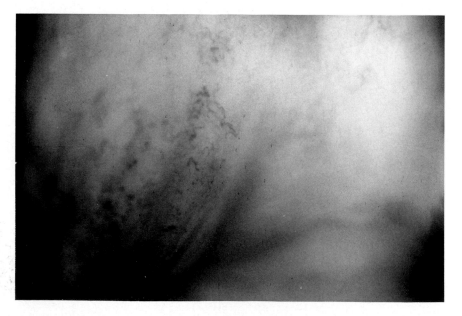

Figure 8-22. Apex of the vagina after postoperative irradiation for endometrial carcinoma. Note the closely packed abnormal blood vessels.

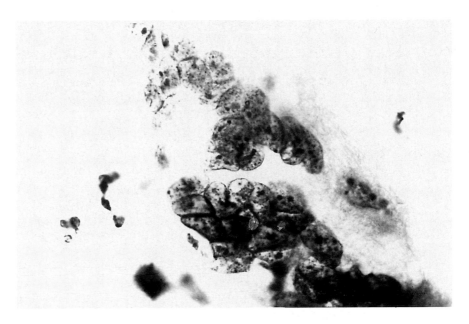

Figure 8-23. Multinucleated cell with abundant vacuolated cytoplasm characteristic of radiation change.

the radiation changes. Postirradiation dysplasia may range from mild to severe. The latter may be difficult to distinguish from recurrent squamous cancer (Figure 8–24). The early appearance of postirradiation dysplasia (within 3 years of therapy) has been associated with a high rate of recurrence of cervical carcinoma. In the long-term follow-up of irradiated patients, however, there is no apparent increase in primary vaginal squamous cell carcinoma compared to control populations.

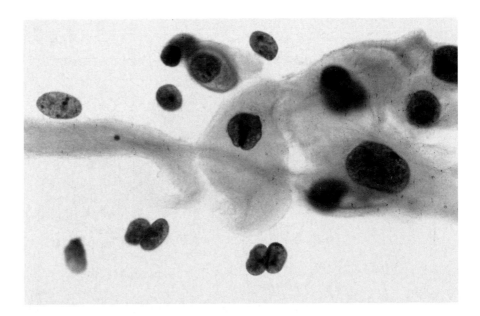

Figure 8-24. Cytology of postirradiation dysplasia. Note nuclear enlargement and hyperchromasia with finely granular chromatin.

TABLE 8-1. VAGINAL INTRAEPITHELIAL NEOPLASIA (VaIN)

Definition	Grade of VaIN
Mild dysplasia	I
Moderate dysplasia	II
Severe dysplasia and carcinoma in situ	III

Vaginal Intraepithelial Neoplasia

Although primary invasive squamous cell carcinoma of the vagina is said to account for 1% to 2% of all genital tract malignancies, the incidence and prevalence of vaginal carcinoma in situ are unknown. Increased use of colposcopy and increased awareness of the "field effect" associated with squamous neoplasia of the female lower genital tract, however, have revised our concepts concerning dysplasia and carcinoma in situ of the vagina.

Most cases of VaIN occur in patients who had a total hysterectomy for cervical intraepithelial neoplastic (CIN) disease. The clinical entity is asymptomatic and is usually detected by routine cytology. Ninety percent of the cases will be found in the upper one third of the vagina. There are several factors that should make one think of VaIN. Patients who have had preinvasive or invasive carcinoma of the cervix, preinvasive or invasive carcinoma of the vulva, prior radiation therapy, HPV infections, cancer chemotherapy, and immunosuppression for either organ transplant or cortisonelike drugs for various medical diseases are all at high risk for developing VaIN.

The classification of vaginal dysplasia and carcinoma in situ is the same as that for the cervix (Table 8-1). Similarly, the cytologic and histologic diagnosis of VaIN depends primarily on the recognition of nuclear abnormalities, including nuclear en-

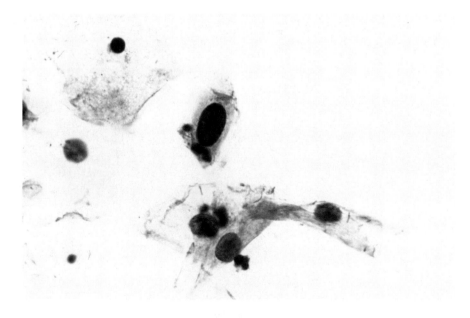

Figure 8-25.   Cytosmear of VaIN III. The cell in the center shows nuclear hyperchromasia and an increased nuclear:cytoplasmic ratio.

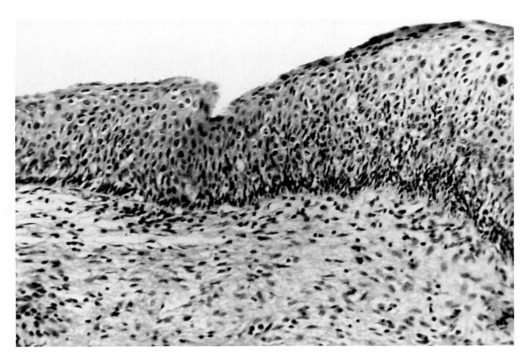

Figure 8-26. Vaginal biopsy with intraepithelial neoplasia grade II. The nuclei of the squamous cells are hyperchromatic with evidence of some cellular maturation in the upper half of the mucosa.

largement, hyperchromasia, and aberrations in chromatin pattern (Figure 8-25). The more severely dysplastic cellular changes are accompanied by a decrease or a loss of cytoplasmic maturation, an increasing nuclear:cytoplasmic ratio, and abnormal mitotic figures. In grade I lesions of VaIN, these abnormalities are confined to the lowest one third of the mucosa; in grade II lesions, they extend to the mid-third; and in grade III lesions they involve the uppermost third (severe dysplasia) or the full thickness of the mucosa (carcinoma in situ). Human papilloma virus related cellular changes, such as nuclear wrinkling and koilocytosis, may be evident in the upper layer of the epithelium, particularly in the less severe degrees of change (ie, VaIN I and II) (Figure 8-26).

Clinically VaIN is usually asymptomatic. Like its counterpart on the cervix, it is usually detected after a routine cytosmear is reported to contain dysplastic squamous cells. Cytology is the most important method for detecting vaginal intraepithelial neoplasia. Hernandez-Linares noted that in 80% of his study group, an abnormal smear was the first clue to the final discovery of the vaginal lesion.

On routine pelvic examination, the findings vary from normal to the presence of leukoplakia or superficial abrasions resulting from insertion of the speculum (related to the diminished intercellular cohesion in dysplastic epithelium). Colposcopic examination, including the use of Lugol's iodine staining of the vagina, will show a diversity of changes that tend to be multifocal. Prior to the application of acetic acid, areas of VaIN are slightly raised, pinkish or white lesions with sharp borders typically located in the fornices of the vagina or adjacent to the edge of the cervix (Figure 8-27, Figure 8-28a, Figure 8-28b). Viewing the lesions at higher magnification, one can appreciate punctation accompanied by variable increases in intercapillary distances, depending on the severity of the lesion (Figure 8-29a, Figure 8-29b, Figure 8-29c, Color Plate 20, Color Plate 21). After the application of 3% acetic acid, the foci of the VaIN assume a grade

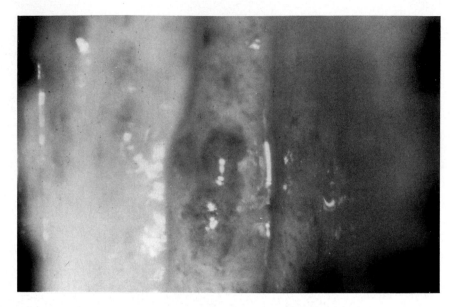

Figure 8-27. Right fornix of the vagina before acetic acid. A red, raised lesion is present that on biopsy revealed VaIN II.

II to III aceto-white appearance interspersed with a coarse papillary punctation; they rarely, if ever, show a mosaic pattern. These lesions characteristically are iodine negative (Figure 8-30).

The treatment of intraepithelial neoplasia is primarily through the use of the carbon dioxide laser or by the application of a 5% Fluorouracil cream (Efudex). These may be used either singly or in combination. The surgical approach of vaginectomy with the inlaying of split-thickness graft is reserved only for those cases in which cures cannot be obtained using the other modalities.

Invasive Carcinoma

When invasion occurs in vaginal squamous neoplasia, a change in the vasculature develops. The vessels become elongated and irregular within the papillary excrescences of raised vaginal lesions. Frequently, these lesions will be ulcerated as well. An invasive adenocarcinoma, due either to metastases or to a primary vaginal tumor, will assume an appearance similar to any invasive malignancy. Atypical blood vessels are the most consistent feature; possibly, the vasculature is somewhat more dilated and coarser than in invasive squamous cell lesions (Figure 8-31, Figure 8-32). One cannot, however, determine the nature of the malignancy colposcopically based on these vascular differences; histologic evaluation is necessary to distinguish these lesions. Adenocarcinoma is described in the chapter concerning the changes related to in utero exposure to DES (*see* Chapter 12). Invasive squamous cell carcinoma has histologic features like those of analogous cervical lesions: various degrees of differentiation, irregular masses and cords of tumor, and, commonly, an accompanying inflammatory response and vascular space invasion. Cytologic findings are, likewise, similar to those of invasive cervical tumors (*see* Chapter 7).

Vaginal Changes Associated with In Utero Exposure to Diethylstilbestrol

Chapter 12 details the effects of exposure to DES on the vagina.

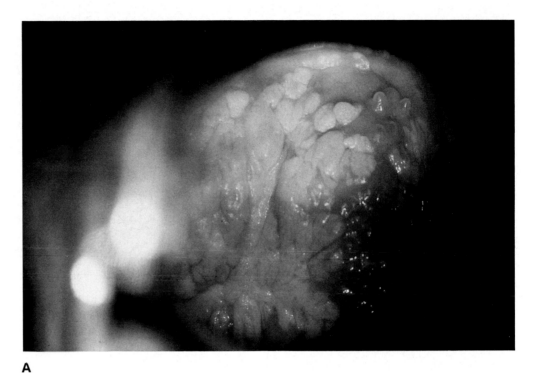

A

B

Figure 8-28.   A. Apex of posthysterectomy vagina after the application of acetic acid. Aceto-white lesions are evident. **B.** Biopsy of Figure 8-28A showing VaIN III. Squamous cells with hyperchromatic nuclei and increased nuclear:cytoplasmic ratio occupy the full thickness of the mucosa in the right half of the photograph.

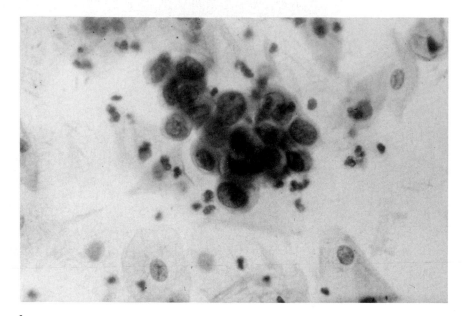

A

B

Figure 8-29. A. Cytosmear with group of cells consistent with VaIN III. **B.** Apex of vagina after hysterectomy for CIN III. Colpophotograph is prior to the application of acetic acid. Note the coarse punctate vessels with increased intercapillary distances. (*Figure continues.*)

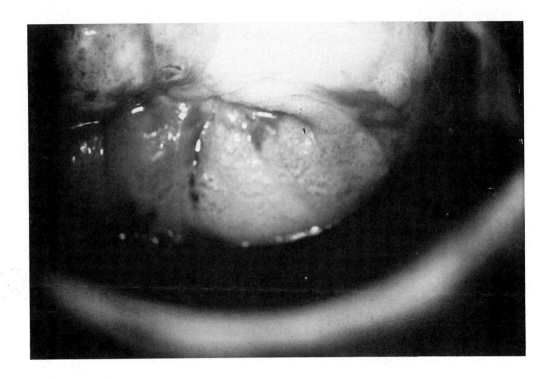

C

Figure 8-29. (continued).   C. Vagina of Figure 8-29B after acetic acid. Note the grade III aceto-white epithelium with punctation. Biopsy revealed VaIN III.

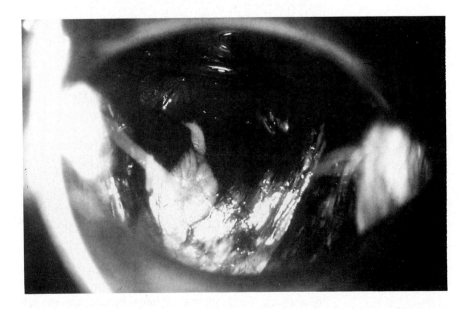

Figure 8-30.   Anterior vaginal wall after Lugol's iodine staining. Note lesions that do not take the stain. Biopsy revealed VaIN III.

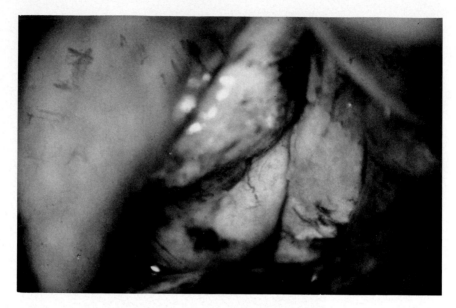

Figure 8-31.   Posterior wall of the vagina of a patient with invasive squamous cell carcinoma of the vagina. Note the prominent abnormal blood vessel.

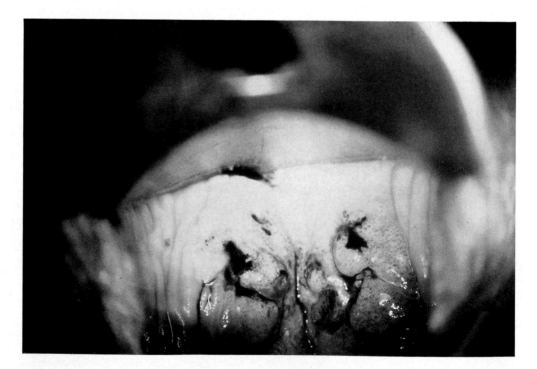

Figure 8-32.   Apex of vagina with metastatic adenocarcinoma of the endometrium 1 year posthysterectomy. Note the coarse punctation and the large, dilated atypical blood vessel.

Chapter 9 | Colposcopy of the Vulva

HISTOLOGY OF THE VULVA

Colposcopic evaluation of the vulva has not proven to be as informative as colposcopy of the cervix and the vagina. This disappointing fact is related to the normal histology of this area, which is lined by a keratinized, stratified squamous epithelium. Although the vulvar epithelium averages only 13 mm in thickness, the prominent surface keratin layer obscures the dermal vasculature (Figure 9-1). Thus, punctation and mosaic patterns are difficult to discern on most of the vulva except for the inner portion of the labia minora and the vestibule, areas in which the keratin layer is thinner. Leukoplakia and aceto-white epithelium are, therefore, the most frequent colposcopic manifestations of vulvar pathology; abnormal blood vessels will be identified when an invasive neoplasm is present. In addition, numerous rugae and papillae are present in the labia minora and near the hymeneal ring. These occasionally fuse and coalesce (Figure 9-2a, 9-2b), and can be misinterpreted as representing human papilloma virus infection (*see* Chapter 10). The urethra, perineum, perianal area, and anus are all considered, colposcopically, to be part of the vulva.

Other histologic features differ from those of the cervix and the vagina. The vulvar epithelium forms rete ridges, and much of the vulva contains hair follicles, sebaceous glands, and apocrine glands (Figure 9-3). The glandular skin appendages become less numerous as the hymeneal ring is approached, but the vestibule contains indigenous mucous glands of two types: the complex tubuloalveolar Bartholin's glands and the simpler minor vestibular glands. Additional mucinous glands (paraurethral or Skene's glands) are located lateral to and alongside the urethra and open adjacent to the urethral meatus.

COLPOSCOPY OF THE VULVA

At colposcopy, application of acetic acid and toluidine blue dye aids in delinating vulvar lesions. The technique of acetic acid application is similar to that used on the cervix and the vagina. To be more effective on the keratinized vulvar skin, the acid must be applied frequently, in large amounts, in a more concentrated form (5%), and be kept in prolonged contact with the epithelial surface. In this way, aceto-white lesions become well defined, and underlying vascular changes (mosaic pattern, punctation) may even become visible, particularly in the labia minora and vestibule (Figures 9-4a, 9-4b, 9-4c,

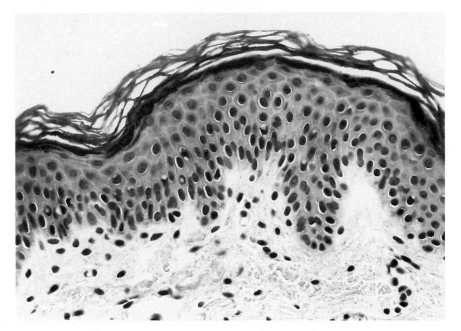

Figure 9-1. Normal skin of vulva. At the surface of the multilayered squamous epithelium, there is keratohyaline granule formation and a surface layer of keratin.

9-4d). The pronounced acidification of the epithelium, however, may interfere with the uptake of toluidine blue if this dye is used subsequently.

Toluidine blue is a nuclear stain; when applied in vivo, it becomes fixed to cell nuclei. To be effective, the toluidine blue must be applied to skin that is completely free of ointments and powders. The dye, applied to the vulva as a 1% aqueous solu-

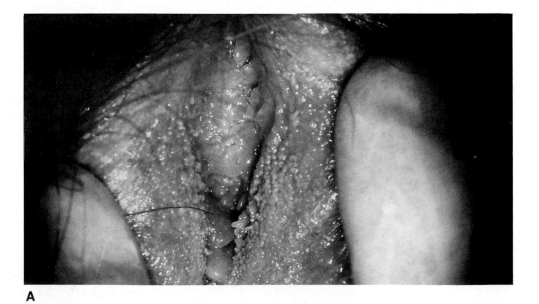

A

Figure 9-2. **A.** Labia minora of the vulva with numerous micropapillae. (*Figure continues.*)

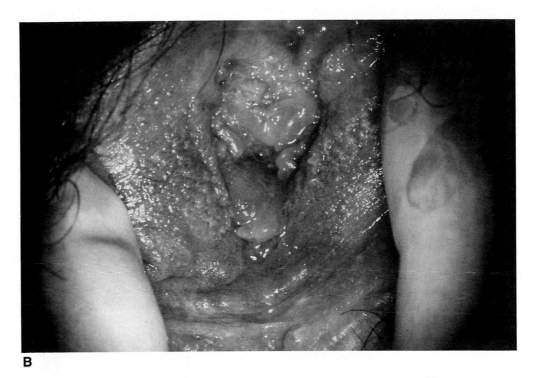

B

Figure 9-2 (continued).   B. Labia minora with fused papillae.

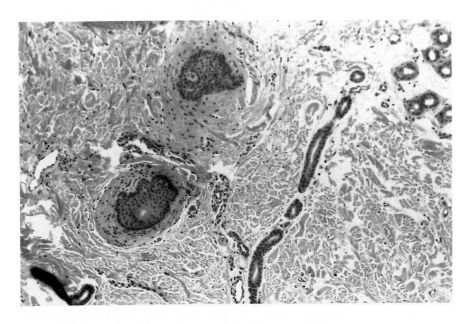

Figure 9-3.   Skin appendages in the dermis of the vulva. On the left side, the rounded structures are hair follicles; on the right, the tubular structures are eccrine sweat ducts.

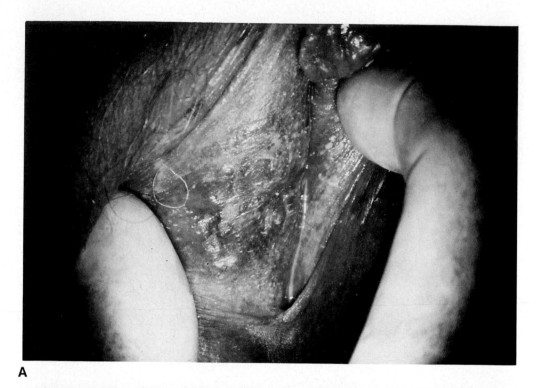

A

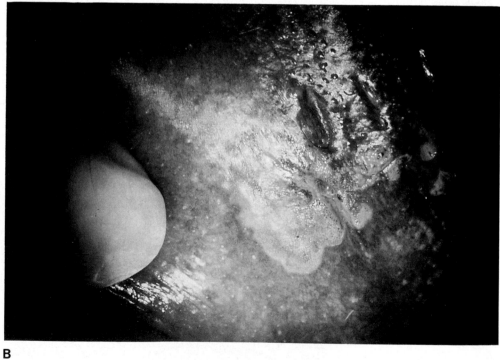

B

Figure 9-4.   A. Labium majus of a 65-year-old patient complaining of pruritus. There is the suggestion of early leukoplakia. **B.** Labium majus after the application of acetic acid. An aceto-white lesion is visible. (*Figure continues.*)

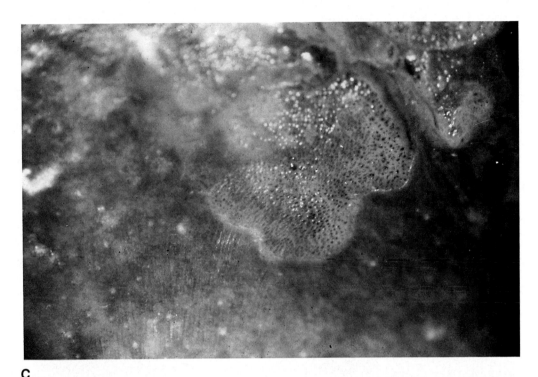

C

D

Figure 9–4 (continued). C. Higher power view of Figure 9–4B. Note the punctation with some increase in the intercapillary distances. **D.** Biopsy of Figure 9–4C showing vulvar intraepithelial neoplasia III. At each end of the photograph, note the capillaries perforating the epithelium and going to the surface to produce the image of punctation.

tion, is kept on the skin surface for two minutes. The vulvar epithelium is then decolorized by washing with 1% acetic acid. On the normal vulva the toluidine blue will be washed away completely by the acetic acid because the surface keratin layer is anucleate. Any condition that results in nucleated cells being present at the skin surface will cause retention of the dye as fine, punctate blue dots that can be readily identified under colposcopic magnification (Figure 9–5, Color Plate 22, Color Plate 23). Erosions and ulcerations will also cause retention of the dye. Nucleated cells at the epithelial surface may be due to the presence of either immature squamous cells or nucleated squames (parakeratosis). Both types of cells are the result of rapid cellular turnover due to a variety of benign and neoplastic conditions. Thus, a positive toluidine blue test is useful for determining areas for biopsy since it defines a focus of abnormal squamous maturation. It does not, however, give any information as to the cause of the abnormality.

BIOPSY OF THE VULVA

The foremost method of evaluating vulvar lesions is microscopic examination of biopsy specimens. Although such specimens are relatively easy to obtain using a variety of instruments, the patient must be prepared by anesthetizing the biopsy site. The use of a topical anesthetic (Hurricane) and the injection of 1% lidocaine by way of a fine 27 gauge dental needle will minimize the discomfort attendant to taking the specimen (Figure 9–6).

The most commonly used biopsy instrument is the Keyes punch, available either as a disposable kit or as reuseable stainless steel instruments (Figure 9–7). Fine tissue forceps and plastic scissors are needed to remove the specimen. Care should be taken not to go too deep or else sutures will be necessary to control the bleeding. A simpler method of retrieving tissue is to use the usual cervical biopsy forceps (Burke or Tischler instruments). A wheal of lidocaine is raised and, with the biopsy forceps, the top of

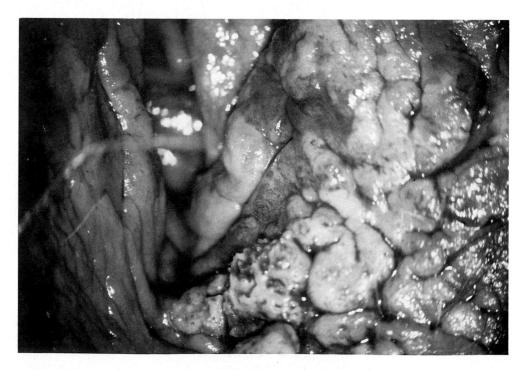

Figure 9–5. Lesion of vulva after the application of toluidine blue and denaturing with 1% acetic acid.

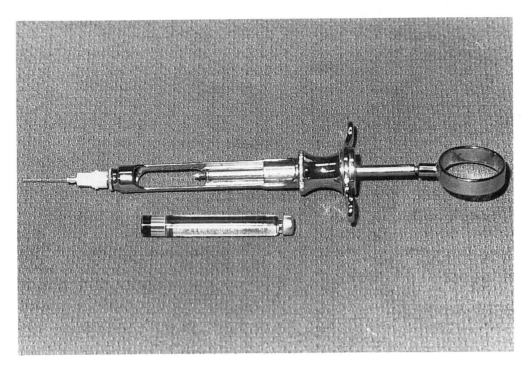

Figure 9-6. Dental syringe with 27 gauge needle. An ampule of local anesthetic is inserted into the barrel of the syringe.

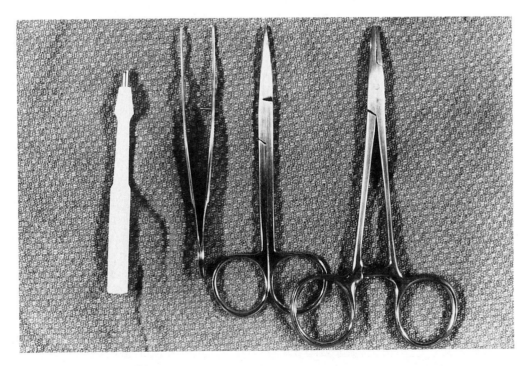

Figure 9-7. Keyes punch set for vulva biopsy. Set includes punch, tissue forceps, scissors, and needle holder.

TABLE 9-1. PROPOSED ISSVD CLASSIFICATION OF VULVAR SQUAMOUS LESIONS [a]

1. Non-neoplastic epithelial disorders (dystrophies)
   a. Squamous cell hyperplasia (formally hyperplastic dystrophy)
   b. Lichen sclerosus
   c. Other dermatoses
2. Vulvar intraepithelial neoplasia (VIN)
   a. VIN I: Mild dysplasia
   b. VIN II: Moderate dysplasia
   c. VIN III: Severe dysplasia and carcinoma in situ
3. Invasive carcinoma

[a]Modification of 1986 proposal.
ISSVD = International Society for the Study of Vulvar Disease.

the wheal is removed (Figures 9–8a, 9–8b, 9–8c). Bleeding will be minimal and can be readily controlled with the application of ferric subsulfate (Monsel's solution).

Histopathologic examination of biopsy specimens from vulvar lesions will identify a spectrum of abnormalities ranging from inflammatory dermatoses, similar to those encountered in extra-genital skin, though premalignant intraepithelial neoplasia and invasive carcinomas. In an attempt to categorize these various pathologic conditions, the International Society for the Study of Vulvar Disease (ISSVD) has proposed a classification system for vulvar lesions (Table 9–1). Some of the more common lesions encountered by the practicing gynecologist are now described.

COMMON VULVAR LESIONS

Condyloma Acuminatum

As on the cervix and the vagina, vulvar condylomas may be exophytic or flat, and they are frequently multiple. Colposcopically, they appear as areas of leukoplakia or aceto-

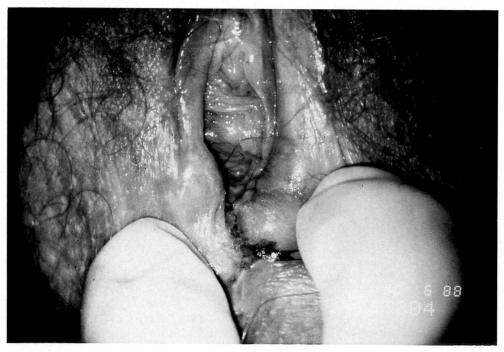

A

Figure 9-8. **A.** Biopsy of vulva; wheal of local anesthetic injected. (*Figure continues.*)

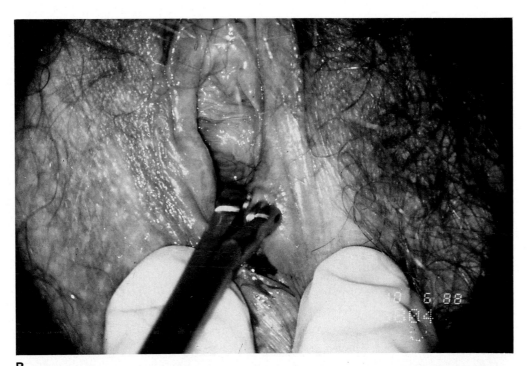

Figure 9–8 (continued). B. Biopsy of vulva; biopsy being taken with a Burke biopsy punch. **C.** Biopsy of vulva; biopsy site.

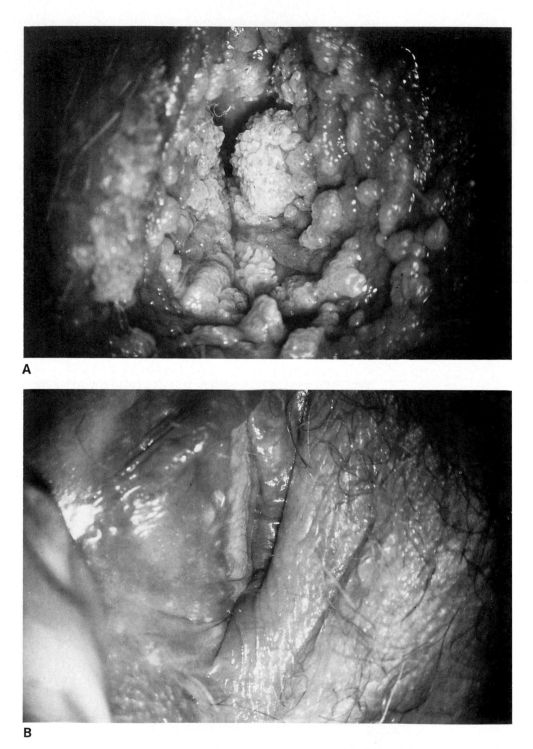

A

B

Figure 9-9.   A. Multiple exophytic condyloma of vulva. **B.** Labia minora after acetic acid with aceto-white change. Biopsy revealed koilocytosis consistent with condyloma.

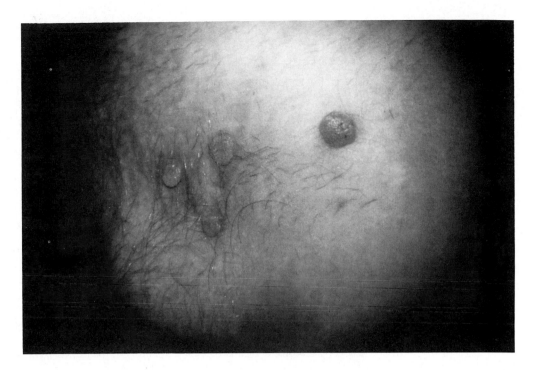

Figure 9-10. Condyloma persisting after podophyllin treatment (*see* Color Plate 24).

white epithelium; however, on the labia minora a fine punctation may also be discerned because of the minimal amount of surface keratin in this area (Figure 9–9a, Figure 9–9b). In patients unsuccessfully treated with podophyllin, the condylomas will often be darker and flatter than usual, with a decrease or absence of the spicules typical of the exophytic lesions (Figure 9–10, Color Plate 24).

Histologically, the findings are the same as those described for the cervix and vagina. True papillary lesions, with prominent fibrovascular cores, are more frequent on the vulva than higher in the genital tract. The microscopic differential diagnosis includes vulvar intraepithelial neoplasia and verrucous carcinoma (*see below*). Use of podophyllin as a therapeutic agent may induce short-term changes in the condyloma that can be detected in the biopsy specimens. These changes include mitotic arrest in metaphase, occasional abnormal mitoses, and nuclear karyorrhexis. These aberrations, however, are rapidly reversible, usually within 1 to 2 weeks after cessation of podophyllin use. To avoid difficulties in the interpretation of the specimens, podophyllin should be discontinued at least 2 weeks prior to biopsy.

Squamous Cell Hyperplasia (Hyperplastic Dystrophy)

The colposcopic appearance of squamous cell hyperplasia (SCH) is a sharply delineated, elevated thickening of the skin with keratinization but without vascular changes (leukoplakia) (Figure 9–11). Microscopically, the features of vulvar SCH are equivalent to lichen simplex chronicus described in other skin sites. The epithelium is thickened secondary to increased layers of benign maturing squamous cells (acanthosis) associated with prominent thickening of the keratin layer (hyperkeratosis) and granular layer (hypergranulosis). Parakeratosis is not typical but may be noted on occasion. Thus, these lesions generally do not stain with toluidine blue. The squamous cell proliferation may be characterized by lengthening of the rete ridges and dermal papillae, similar to that noted in psoriasis. The superficial dermis is sclerotic and contains a variable amount of mononuclear inflammation (Figure 9–12). Squamous cell hyperplasia is not associated with cellular atypia and is not a premalignant condition.

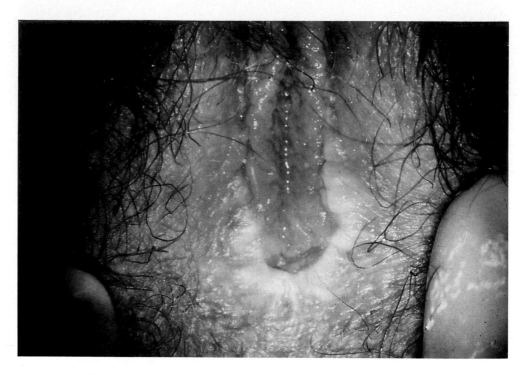

Figure 9-11. Leukoplakia of perineum and introitus (*see* Figure 9-12).

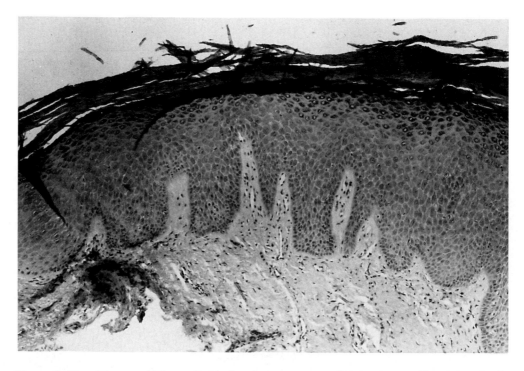

Figure 9-12. Biopsy of Figure 9-11 showing squamous thickening and hyperkeratosis of the epithelium.

Lichen Sclerosus

Lichen sclerosus (LS) may occur at any skin site and at any age but it characteristically develops on the vulva in middle-aged and older white females. On the vulva, LS tends to form areas of flat or papular white epithelium. The surface is often shiny, with a crinkled appearance (Figure 9–13). Diminution of the underlying dermis and subcutaneous tissue may lead to atrophy of the labia and constriction of the introitus. Areas of leukoplakia suggest an accompanying SCH. Histologically, LS has three characteristic features:

1. Edema (early stage of LS) and hyalization (late stage) of collagen in the dermis.
2. Vacuolization of the epidermal basal cells.
3. Mononuclear inflammation located deep to the dermal changes.

In the early phases of LS, the epidermis is of normal thickness, but over time it becomes atrophic (Figure 9–14). Lichen sclerosus may exist alone or be associated with other lesions such as SCH or dysplasia. By itself, LS has no malignant potential; however, accompanying areas of biopsy-proven dysplasia must be appropriately treated.

The etiology of LS is unknown. The affected tissue is reversibly atrophic and has normal maturation potential. Friedrich and his co-workers have demonstrated that women with vulvar LS had significantly decreased serum levels of dihydrotestosterone and androstenedione. Based on this, the usual treatment for this condition is the application of a 2% testosterone proprionate ointment, which significantly increases the serum levels of both dihydrotestosterone and testosterone. In addition, testosterone has a stimulating effect on the skin and skin derivatives.

The 2% ointment is mixed by the pharmacist by adding 30 mL of testosterone proprionate in sesame oil (100 mgm/cc) with 120 gms of white petrolatum. The resultant ointment is applied twice a day for 6 months. Once limitation of symptoms has occurred, a maintenance dose once a week is necessary. The patient is alerted to the possibility of virilization (hair growth, deepening of the voice, enlargement of the clitoris).

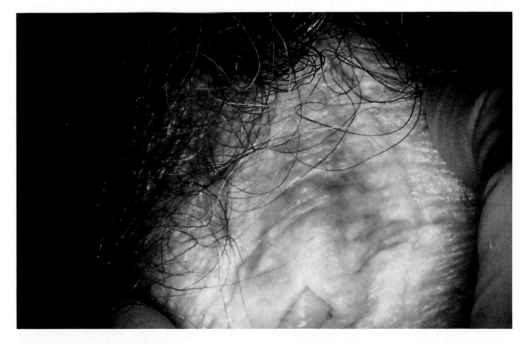

Figure 9-13. Periclitoral area of a 60-year-old patient with pruritus. Note the crinkled, whitish epithelium.

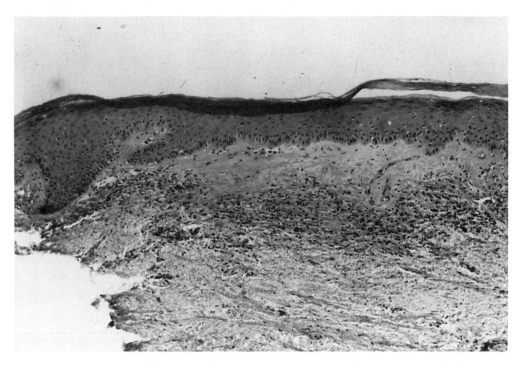

Figure 9-14. Biopsy of Figure 9-13 showing the characteristic findings of LS. The superficial dermis is homogenized and degenerated. Beneath it is a band of mononuclear inflammatory cells.

Increased libido with erotic dreams may be especially troublesome for elderly, postmenopausal women. If any of the symptoms described above occur, the testosterone ointment should be stopped. A substitute ointment using medroxyprogesterone (Provera) can be substituted for the testosterone. Although not as efficacious as the testosterone ointment, it does provide relief for some patients. Laser ablation and surgical excision should be considered a last resort in extreme cases, as they usually afford no relief.

Vulvar Intraepithelial Neoplasia

Vulvar intraepithelial neoplasia (VIN) is seen most often in women during their reproductive years. Fifty percent of cases are under the age of 40, and the mean age is 35 to 40 years. Twenty-five to fifty percent of the lesions are associated with condyloma acuminatum and 30% of the patients have cervical intraepithelial neoplasia (CIN) or vaginal intraepithelial neoplasia (VaIN). Thus, the diagnosis of VIN dictates the evaluation of the cervix and vagina by colposcopy. More than 50% of the patients may be asymptomatic; the rest of the patients usually complain of pruritus and a very small number will note some type of lesion in the vulvar area. The lesions of VIN are most often found on the inferior margins of the labia majora and minora, on the perineal body, in the periclitoral area, and around the anus.

Colposcopically, the appearance of VIN may mimic that of SCH or LS, so that biopsy evaluation of all such lesions is mandatory. Vulvar intraepithelial neoplasia, which may be uni- or multifocal, may present as leukoplakia or aceto-white epithelium (Figure 9-15, Figure 9-16). Vascular changes are generally inconspicuous except for VIN on the labia minora, in which case punctation or mosaic pattern may be evident (*see* Figures 9-4c; Figures 9-17a, 9-17b). High-grade lesions (VIN II or VIN III) may be variegated, with areas of brown, red, blue, and white coloration (Color Plate 25, Color Plate 26).

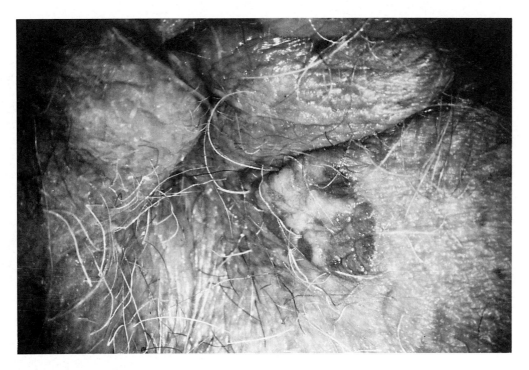

Figure 9-15. Lesion in the perianal area. The lesion has leukoplakic change and bluish discoloration (*see* Color Plate 25).

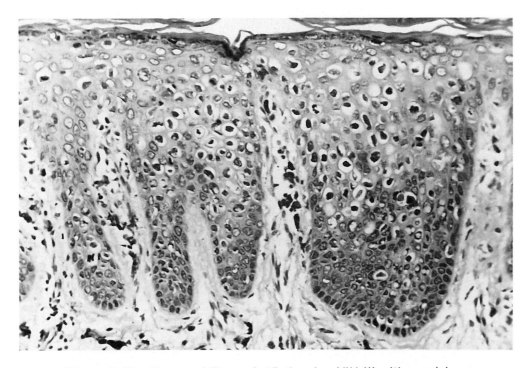

Figure 9-16. Biopsy of Figure 9-15 showing VIN III with condyloma.

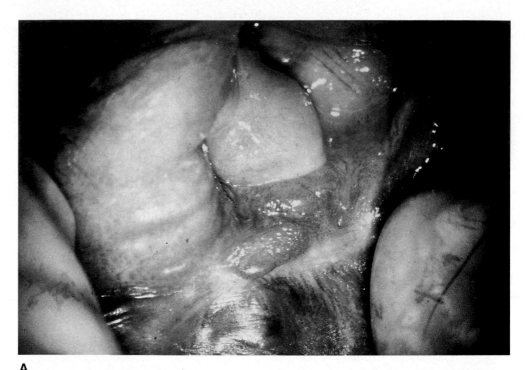

A

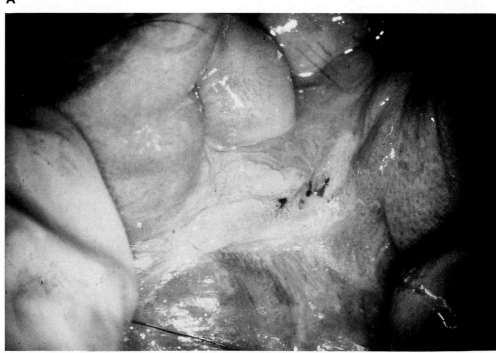

B

Figure 9-17. **A.** Introitus of vulva prior to acetic acid. Note area with asperities. **B.** Lesion in Figure 9-17A after acetic acid. Note aceto-white area with punctation.

The histologic features of VIN grades I, II, and III are identical to their counterparts on the cervix and the vagina with the exception that parakeratosis, and on occasion, keratinization, may be noted with VIN (Figure 9–18).

The treatment of VIN traditionally involved surgery. With the advent of the use of the carbon dioxide laser in gynecology, however, this has become the method of choice in treating this disease. The "skinning vulvectomy" can be done as an alternative surgical approach.

Invasive Carcinoma

Invasive carcinoma of the vulva comprises 4% of primary malignancy of the female genital tract. The average age is 60 years; however, it can be seen in younger patients. This is especially true in those patients who have had some form of a prior granulomatous lesion. The lesions of invasive carcinoma may be asymptomatic; when symptoms and signs are present they include pruritus, pain, bleeding, or palpable lesion.

The diagnosis of invasive carcinoma generally does not require colposcopic examination. The lesions are usually raised, may be red or white, and are typically ulcerated (Figures 9–19, 9–20a, 9–20b, 9–20c). Colposcopically, however, one can find the usual criteria of invasion: areas of necrosis that have a yellowish appearance and, most importantly, abnormal blood vessels. The value of the colposcope in identifying these lesions is most evident in the early stages of the disease when patients are frequently being treated for other entities with topical creams. Colposcopy at this time may identify

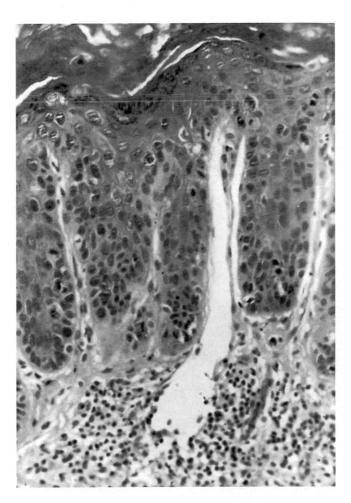

Figure 9–18. Biopsy of Figure 9–17B showing VIN III.

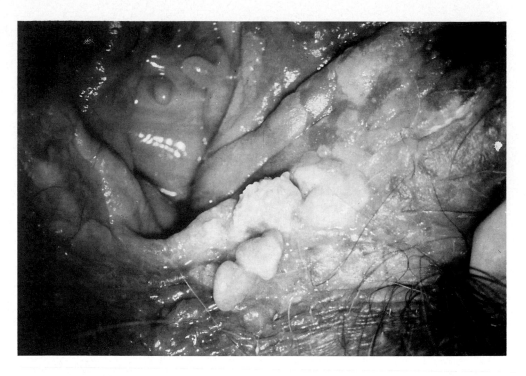

Figure 9–19.   Raised white lesion that has been treated for 6 months as a condyloma. Biopsy of the superior reddish area revealed invasive carcinoma.

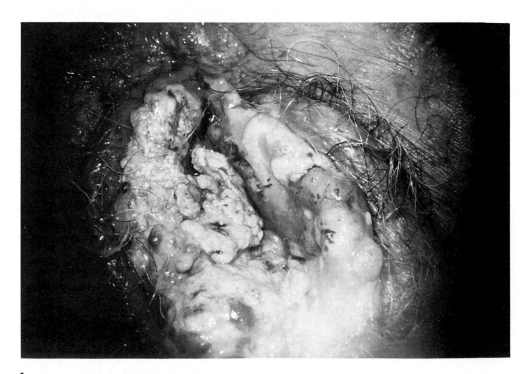

A

Figure 9–20.   **A.** Obvious, ulcerated exophytic carcinoma of the vulva. (*Figure continues.*)

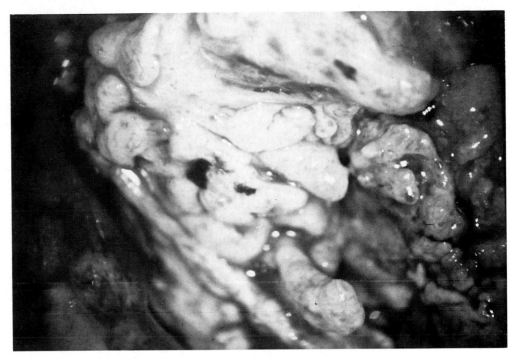

B

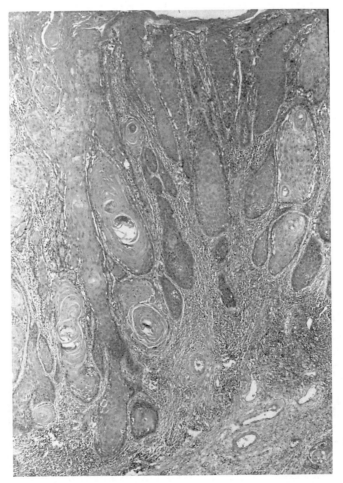

C

Figure 9–20 (continued).   B. Higher powered view of Figure 9–20A showing atypical blood vessels. **C.** Biopsy of lesion of Figure 9–20B showing invasive squamous carcinoma. Nodules of well-differentiated keratinizing squamous cells extend deep into the dermis.

areas that are different from the obvious and that, on biopsy, will show evidence of an invasive squamous cell carcinoma. In addition, colposcopy may be helpful in determining the extent of involvement of the vulva and aid in delineating the margins of the surgical specimen to be taken.

The basic evaluation of vulvar lesions, as already noted, requires biopsy. Because many vulvar lesions are multifocal, the magnification of the colposcope is needed for adequate identification of all lesions. Many lesions of diverse etiology may appear similar even under colposcopic magnification; biopsy is therefore mandatory for ruling out neoplastic disease. Biopsy will lead to correct diagnosis and proper therapy.

Figure 9–21 is an allogram outlining a proposed method of investigating a suspicious vulvar lesion.

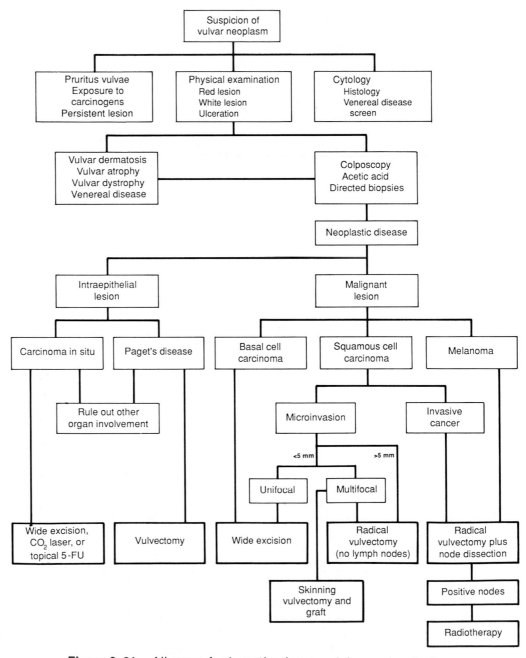

Figure 9–21.   Allogram for investigating suspicious vulvar lesions.

Chapter 10 | Colposcopy and the Human Papilloma Virus

INTRODUCTION

A marked increase in the incidence and prevalence of venereal warts of the lower genital tract has occurred in the past two decades. The Centers for Disease Control has documented a 45% increase in this diagnosis over the past 15 years; currently there are over 2 million consultations per year concerning this disease in the United States. The peak prevalence of venereal warts is in young women of childbearing age, most women being between the ages of 15 and 30. Data on the true prevalence of these infections are difficult to obtain because of the inability to culture the etiologic agent and the lack of a serologic test to determine exposure. The presently available tests, including the recently developed molecular biology techniques, have serious limitations to their use in the epidemiologic and clinical setting. No single diagnostic test reliably detects all stages of human papilloma virus (HPV) infection or HPV-associated disease at each genital site.

ETIOLOGY

The etiologic agent of venereal warts is the HPV, a member of the papoaviruses family. Human papilloma viruses are small DNA viruses that have similar ultrastructure features on electron microscopy. The papoaviruses include the papilloma virus of rabbits (Shope), the polyomavirus of humans, and the simian vacuolating virus of monkeys.

Viruses are obligatory intracellular parasites that contain only one type of nucleic acid, either DNA or RNA. Thus, they are broadly classified as either DNA or RNA viruses. The nucleic acid core of the virus is surrounded by a protein coat called the capsid, which is composed of repeating units of polypeptides called capsomeres. The capsid acts as a protective coat that stabilizes the virus outside the cell and also aids in virus absorption into and, probably, penetration of the host cell. The nucleic acid core that carries all of the genetic information for the replication of the virus and the capsid constitutes the mature virus particle, called the virion. Whereas the Herpes virus is a very complex virus, the HPV is rather simple, containing a single strand of DNA. The characteristics of the HPV are:

1. The diameter is 55 nm.
2. It has a symmetrical capsid.
3. There are 72 capsomeres.
4. The molecular weight is 5×10^6 daltons.

Reproduction of the Human Papilloma Virus

Because viruses do not contain the equipment for reproduction, they require living cells for multiplication. The host cell, activated by the viral genome, supplies energy and precursor substances for viral replication. Most infections are sexually transmitted because of the innoculation of the virus into the new host at sites of microtrauma, but innoculation can also occur during the passage of the newborn through an infected maternal lower genital tract. The HPV virion penetrates the squamous epithelium to reach the basal layer. The virus penetrates the basal cells by first attaching its capsid to the cell membrane, then by penetrating the membrane. Within the cytoplasm, the virion is uncoated and the viral genome is then transported to the nucleus in which translation and transcription occur, thus producing various virus-specific proteins. In about 60% of infected cells, complete viral replication occurs: new genetic material is synthesized, and a new capsid coat is assembled into which the genes are inserted, and the new virions escape from the cell either by cell lysis or budding. In about 40% of infected cells, however, viral replication is aborted or incomplete. No new viral DNA or capsid protein is produced, probably because of a lack of host cell function. Rather, the DNA of the original, infective virion is inserted into the host cell genome and is then replicated with the cell. The infective virus does not lyse the host cell. The infection may thus remain latent, but in some patients, the interaction of virus and host nucleus causes transformation of the cell accompanied by loss of certain cellular responses to environmental control. Among these is the loss of mitotic inhibition so that cells continue to divide above the basal zone.

HISTOLOGY OF THE HUMAN PAPILLOMA VIRUS

Productive HPV infection of squamous mucosa results in epithelial proliferation producing characteristic histologic features. There is an increased number of cell layers (acanthosis), particularly involving the parabasal cells. The proliferating mucosa may remain flat or assume a papillary configuration. Continued DNA synthesis by parabasal and intermediate cells is reflected microscopically by a mild nuclear hyperchromatism, dyskaryosis, and delayed surface maturation. In the upper layers, the late events in the viral life cycle (those concerned with actual viral replication) produce a characteristic cytopathic effect called koilocytosis.

A large proportion of exposed individuals will remain latently infected for a long time. Until recently, demonstration of the virus in such patients has been hampered by inadequate technology. It is impossible to grow the virus in tissue culture, although there have been attempts to grow it on the renal cortex; this may be of great value in the future. Ultrastructural and immunocytochemical techniques can only detect complete virions, and thus, are not helpful in determining latent infection. DNA hybridization however, can detect HPV DNA sequences within the nuclei of otherwise normal cells, thereby permitting analysis of both latent and overt infection and the classification of cases by genotype. To date, more than 50 distinct genotypes of HPV have been described. Each of the HPV genotypes has a predilection for a limited number of mucosal sites and is associated with a particular set of clinical-pathologic entities. Of the 50 plus currently characterized HPV types, 12 have been associated with lesions of the genital tract. Of the more prevalent types, genotypes 6 and 11 are associated with squamous proliferations of low malignant potential, whereas genotypes 16, 18, 31, 33, and possibly 41, have been associated with the development of carcinomas of the lower genital tract. For example, 80% to 90% of cervical carcinomas contain DNA from HPV 16, 18, or 33.

Human papilloma viral infections begin in the basal layer of the epithelium, although no changes are evident on light microscopy. Viral DNA replication occurs in the proliferating basal and parabasal cells, but structural capsid proteins are not detected. It has been speculated that the basal cell proliferation is due to early gene function, resulting in the synthesis of nonstructural viral proteins that may either stimulate host cell proliferation directly or repress mechanisms controlling proliferation. Immediately above the parabasal zone, the cells begin to mature and differentiate, with the cytoplasm becoming more abundant and eosinophilic because of keratin synthesis. Late gene expression, manifested by the production of viral structure proteins, is detected in these cells as nuclear staining for HPV capsid protein by immunocytochemical techniques. The detection of intranuclear viral particles in these cells on electron microscopic examination indicates complete viral assembly. Because viral DNA may be present in the lesion without synthesis of the structural viral proteins necessary for encapsidation, negative results on ultrastructural or immunocytochemical examinations do not necessarily exclude the presence of HPV. In contrast, late gene expression is necessary for the virus to be infectious and assembly of complete virions can be determined by electron microscopy or immunocytochemistry.

In intraepithelial dysplastic lesions, HPV DNA generally exists in a nonintegrated form within the nucleus of the proliferating cells. Development of invasive carcinomas, however, is associated with integration of HPV DNA into the host genome.

DIAGNOSIS OF HUMAN PAPILLOMA VIRUS

The diagnosis of HPV associated exophytic lesions (condylomata) of the vulva, vagina, and cervix requires no great expertise and no special tests. Confirmation that intraepithelial neoplasia is not present in condylomas should be made by biopsy. Some condylomas may be confused with true malignant lesions because of their associated vascular changes (to be discussed in the following section on the consideration of the colposcopic appearance of HPV).

The subclinical HPV lesions in the vagina and cervix are usually detected by cytology. The two characteristic findings in cytosmears are atypical perakeratotic cells and koilocytes, the latter being virtually pathognomonic of HPV infections. Koilocytes are superficial or intermediate squamous cells that are characterized by the presence of a large perinuclear halo of clear cytoplasm. The peripheral cytoplasm is very dense and stains irregularly, exhibiting a bluish-green color or a dense fuscia-red reaction. The nuclei may become vesicular or be quite dense, hyperchromatic, and pyknotic. Binucleation is frequent, and multinucleation may be seen (Figure 10–1a, Figure 10–1b). The nuclear membrane is wrinkled so that the nucleus has a "raisin" appearance. Atypical perakeratotic cells are small keratinized cells with enlarged, very dense, and sometimes pyknotic, nuclei. The cytoplasm is usually refractile and orange. They occasionally exfoliate in tridimensional aggregates made up of several layers, or they may occur singly as minature squamous cells.

COLPOSCOPY OF HUMAN PAPILLOMA VIRAL GENITAL INFECTION

There are multiple classifications for the colposcopic appearances of HPV infections in the lower genital tract. One of the earliest was proposed by Meisels, Roy, and Fortin, who divided condyloma into the following classes:

1. Exophytic or florid.
2. Early or spiked.
3. Flat or inverted.

Other classifications have used the terms "cerebriform" lesions, "subclinical wart virus

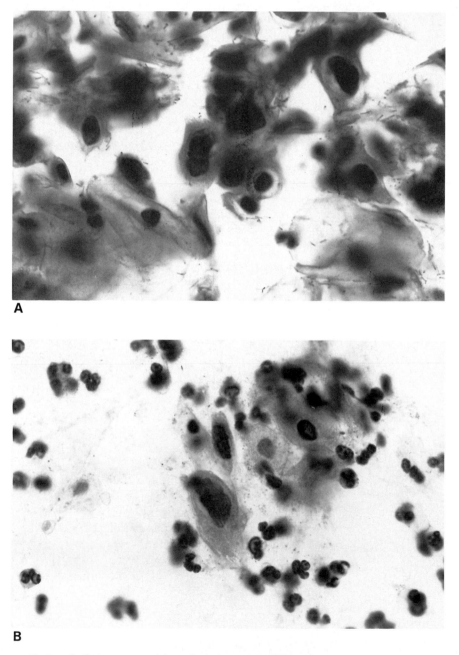

A

B

Figure 10-1.   A. Cytosmear with cells infected by HPV. Note the prominent perinuclear clearing of cytoplasm (koilocytosis). **B.** Cytosmear showing cervical intraepithelial neoplasia with condyloma. Note that atypical cells in the center are binucleated with perinuclear clearing of cytoplasm.

infection," or "subclinical papilloma infection (SPI)," and even the term "condylomatous vaginitis" (Figure 10–2). The flat or inverted condyloma is most frequently designated as the subclinical wart virus infection. Meisel's classification system, with modifications when applied to specific organs, seems to be the most practical.

Exophytic or Florid Condyloma Acuminatum

The colposcopic diagnosis of these lesions, which can also be detected with the naked eye, is usually easy (*see* Figures 8–9, 9–9a; Figures 10–3, 10–4, 10–5). The epithelium has a thick white surface with fingerlike projections showing irregular surface contours. Visualization of a regular capillary loop in each of these projections is the most reliable diagnostic feature and is best seen after the acetic acid has worn off. Occasionally, an exophytic invasive cancer has fingerlike projections resembling those of a florid condyloma. The vascular pattern in the carcinoma, however, will be highly atypical, and the projections will vary in size and coalesce with one another.

Early or Spiked Condyloma

The early or spiked condyloma is not usually seen with the naked eye. It has an irregular surface containing tiny spikes of tissue, called "asperities," which are fingerlike projections that reflect the light from the colposcope (*see* Figure 8–13; Figure 10–6). Usually, no capillary loops are seen in the asperities but punctation may be present in the intervening epithelium. The surface is irregular, and the border between it and the normal tissue may be sharp. These lesions may be difficult to distinguish from CIN.

Flat or Inverted Condyloma

Most HPV infections of the lower genital tract are flat, aceto-white lesions (*see* Figures 5–23b, 8–11, 9–9b; Figures 10–7, 10–8). As a general rule, they are impossible to differentiate from intraepithelial neoplasia (*see* Figures 6–8a, 6–8b, 6–8c). Mosaicism and punctation may be present, but they are usually of the fine, grade I type. Asperities

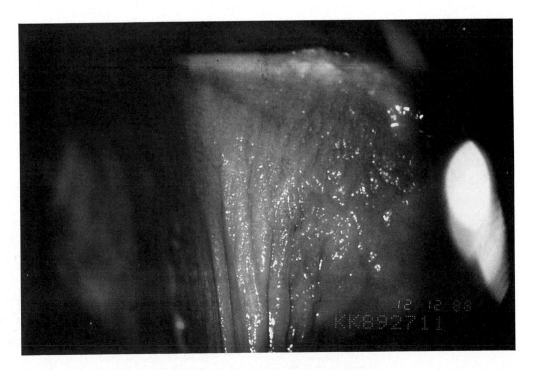

Figure 10–2. Condylomatous vaginitis.

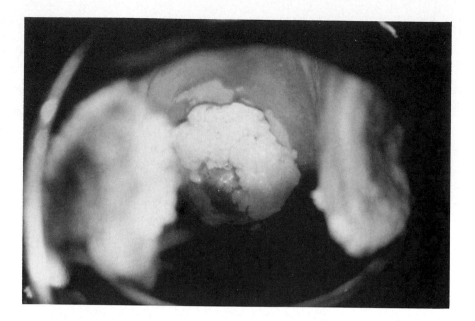

Figure 10-3. Exophytic condyloma of cervix (*see* Figure 10-9A, Figure 10-9B).

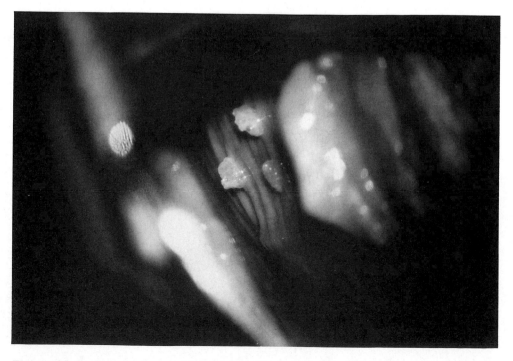

Figure 10-4. Exophytic condyloma of vaginal wall (*see* Figure 8-8, Figure 8-10).

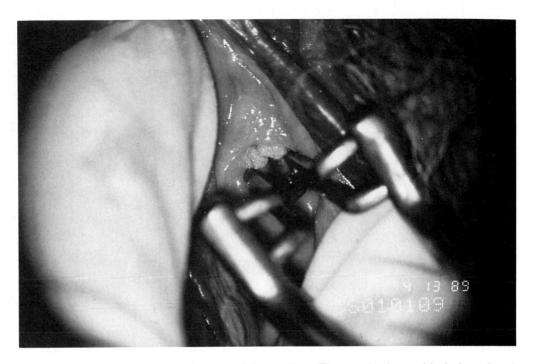

Figure 10-5. Exophytic condyloma of the urethra. The urethral canal is being visualized by means of an endocervical speculum.

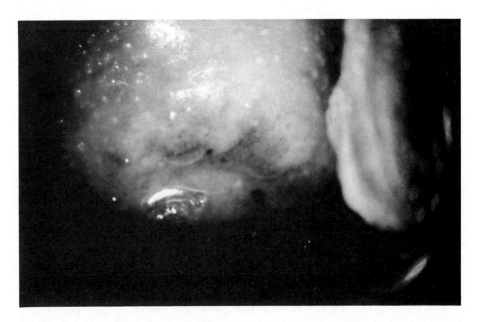

Figure 10-6. Asperities on the surface of the cervix. Biopsy revealed koilocytosis.

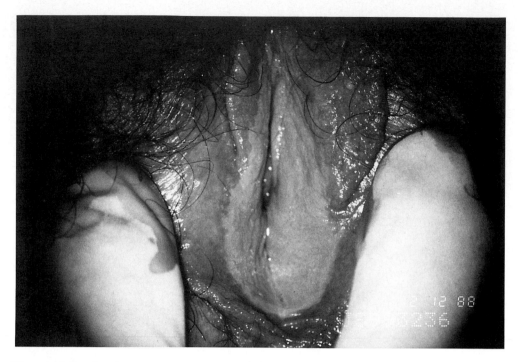

Figure 10–7. Labia minora after application of acetic acid. Note the wide aceto-white involvement of the area.

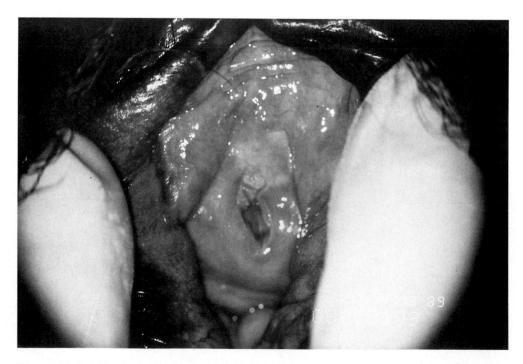

Figure 10–8. Urethra after application of acetic acid. Note the aceto-white changes on the meatus.

may be found in parts of the lesion, and sometimes a cerebriform appearance is identified. If coarse vascular patterns are found, intraepithelial neoplasia should be suspected. In an attempt to differentiate HPV infection from CIN, Reid has advocated the use of Lugol's iodine staining and a colposcopic grading system having four signs:

1. Lesion color.
2. Margin.
3. Vascular pattern.
4. Appearance on iodine staining.

Scores of 0 to 2 are very predictive of a minor lesion (HPV or CIN I). Scores of 3 to 5 usually indicate a middle grade lesion (CIN II). A score of 6 to 8 usually denotes a significant degree of intraepithelial neoplasia (CIN II to III). Reid and Campion, using this particular type of scoring, state that they had a 90% correlation between the colposcopic image and the histologic diagnosis within one grade of histologic severity.

PATHOLOGY

The exophytic or papillomatous lesions, which are uncommon on the cervix but common in the vagina or on the vulva, are characterized by parakeratosis, acanthosis, and papillomatosis (*see* Figures 8–8, 8–10; Figures 10–9a, 10–9b). Koilocytosis is visible in

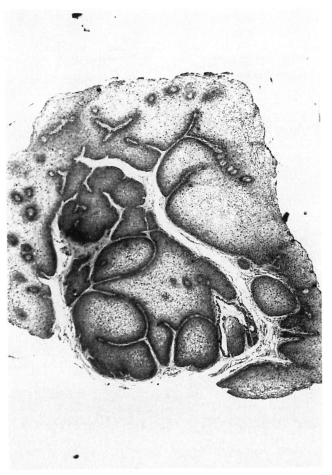

Figure 10–9. A. Low power photomicrograph of exophytic condyloma with acanthosis and papillary fronds cut in cross section. *(Figure continues.)*

A

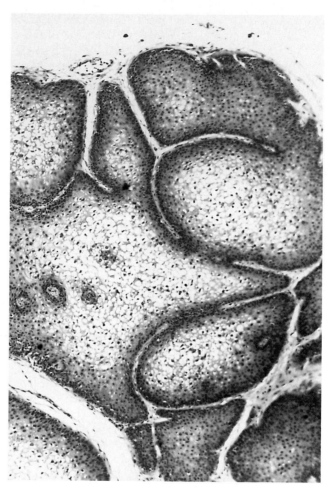

Figure 10-9 (continued). B. Higher power view of Figure 10-9A; the majority of the squamous cells show perinuclear halos (koilocytosis). The basal layer is normal.

B

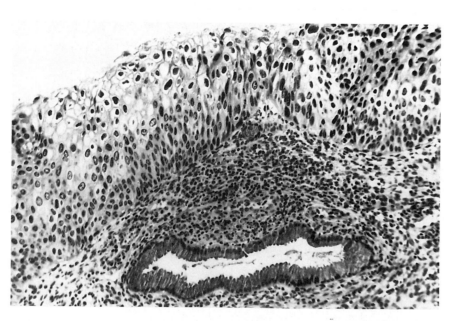

Figure 10-10. Biopsy of atypical condyloma (CIN grade I). The superficial squamous cells show koilocytosis and HPV-related nuclear changes. The basal layers are slightly enlarged and the nuclei are mildly hyperchromatic.

the upper epithelial layers. In the so-called flat condyloma, the basal layers preserve a normal polarization of cells. The papillae of connective tissue become elongated and widened. Small undulations or spikes may appear on the surface of flat condylomas. These spikes, which are formed by blood vessels surrounded by stroma pushing upwards through the epithelium, correspond to asperities observed during colposcopy. The intermediate and superficial layers contain many koilocytes that contrast with the deeper cells having dense and abundant cytoplasm. The nuclei of the intermediate and superficial cells are frequently irregular in shape, vesicular or hyperchromatic, and often multinucleated. These flat lesions represent the most frequent pattern of HPV infection in the cervix, vagina, and vulva (*see* Figure 8–12, Figure 9–9b).

A subgroup of condylomatous lesions, described as the "atypical condyloma," is very confusing and raises many questions in regard to therapy. These lesions show HPV features but have very marked nuclear atypia, so that it is sometimes difficult to differentiate these atypical condylomas from CIN I. The tissue sections must be carefully inspected for the diagnostic features of condyloma: smudged chromatin, perinuclear halos, low nuclear:cytoplasmic ratio, and regularity of the deep epithelial layers (Figure 10–10).

Chapter 11 | Colposcopy and Pregnancy

INTRODUCTION

Because most women at risk of developing cervical carcinoma become pregnant, the best way of screening for this disease is to obtain a cytosmear from all women at the time of their first prenatal visit. The logic behind this approach relates to the fact that the peak prevalence of precancerous conditions of the cervix occurs in the 25- to 35-year age group, which is also the decade of maximum childbearing.

The prevalence of women with abnormal cytology during pregnancy is between 3% and 4%. The incidence of cervical carcinoma among pregnant women is variable in different reports, from a minimum of 1 in 10,000 pregnancies to a maximum of 13 per 10,000 pregnancies. Large maternity hospitals have an average incidence of one carcinoma per 25,000 gestations. One percent of women with carcinoma of the uterine cervix are pregnant at the time of diagnosis.

In general, pregnancy in patients with carcinoma of the cervix occurs only in the early stages of cancer development, because conception is hindered or prevented by a tumor mass. Thus, for patients who present with an abnormal smear during pregnancy, it is imperative to rule out invasive disease that may still be early and localized.

THE PREGNANT CERVIX

In order to evaluate the pregnant cervix, an understanding of the physiologic and histologic changes that occur during pregnancy is necessary. In pregnancy, the diameter of the cervix may increase tenfold, a change usually accompanied by cyanosis and softening because of increased cervical vascularity, edema, and tissue hyperplasia. The vaginal walls also show signs of these tissue changes; they become lax and redundant, a feature that may interfere with the normal visualization of the cervix (Figure 11–1). The epithelium also becomes thicker, and the vaginal tube lengthens.

Histology

Histologically, the stromal edema and increased vascularity are accompanied by acute inflammation. Just prior to labor, collagen breakdown occurs, allowing cervical dilatation. Stromal decidualization occurs in about 30% of pregnant women (Figure 11–2). Endocervical mucinous epithelium proliferates, forming polypoid projections and undergoing squamous metaplasia (microglandular hyperplasia). As a result, there is an increased production of thick, tenacious mucus that not only seals the endocervical canal but may also interfere with adequate visualization of the cervix (Figure 11–3).

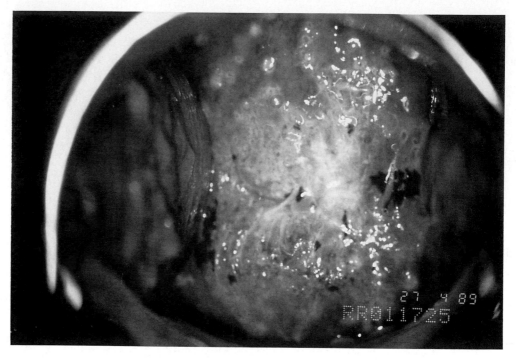

Figure 11–1. A cervix at 25 weeks' gestation. Note that the side walls of the vagina balloon in, making visualization of the cervix difficult.

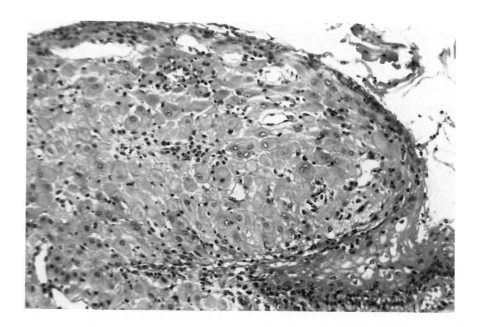

Figure 11–2. Decidualized stroma in cervical biopsy of pregnant female.

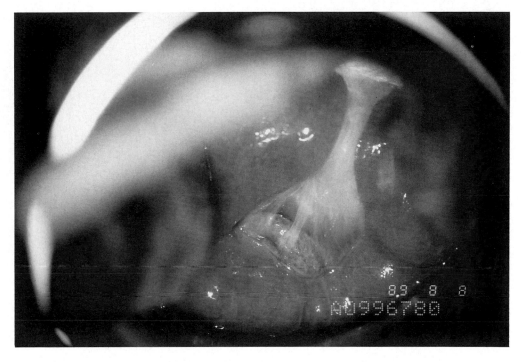

Figure 11-3. Cervix at 28 weeks of gestation. Note the tenacious mucus.

Physiology

Physiologically, two processes result from the high estrogen content of pregnancy. First, there is a rearrangement of the cervical mesenchymal elements and ground substance resulting in an eversion of the endocervical canal that brings it into the lowered pH milieu of the vagina. The extent of this eversion depends primarily on parity, because eversion is more common in the primiparous patient.

A second process develops as a result of the exposure of the everted columnar epithelium to the vaginal environment: squamous metaplasia will occur (as already discussed in Chapters 3 and 4). Squamous metaplasia is most prevalent and extensive in the first pregnancy. The primiparous cervix in the early part of the first trimester is composed of large areas of columnar epithelium that have not undergone squamous metaplasia. During the latter weeks of the first trimester, endocervical eversion and the metaplastic process commence simultaneously; very rapidly, areas of individual columnar villi fuse and become recognizable as distinct islands of immature metaplastic tissue in a sea of columnar epithelium (Figure 11–4). During the second trimester the metaplastic process becomes more active, and the resulting squamous epithelium appears over larger areas as a smooth, opaque covering. In the third trimester the squamous metaplasia continues, although fusion of the individual metaplastic islands and tongues of tissue has normally ceased by the 34th to 36th week. Eversion of the endocervical epithelium continues throughout pregnancy and is more marked during the second and early third trimester than in the first trimester.

During pregnancy, the multiparous cervix undergoes, to a limited extent, most of the epithelial changes described for the primipara. The development of metaplastic squamous epithelium, however, occurs predominantly in the last trimester in contrast to the primipara, in whom it is maximal in the second and early third trimester. In the multipara, eversion is most likely to occur in the last trimester. The external os of the multipara tends to open and gape as pregnancy progresses.

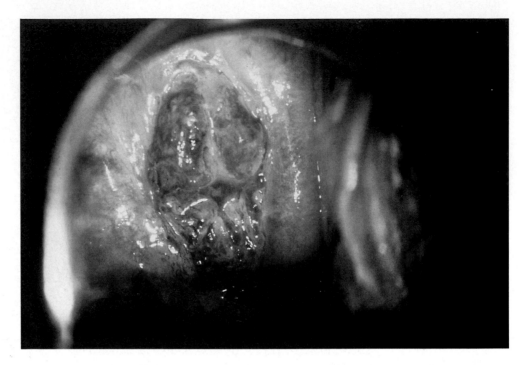

Figure 11-4. Everted cervix at 16 weeks' gestation. Note the areas of metaplasia in the columnar epithelium.

Cytology

The cytologic changes during pregnancy may be somewhat difficult to interpret. Progesterone's effect is prominent, with a marked preponderance of intermediate cells; cytolysis and squamous metaplasia are also evident. In addition, characteristic boat-shaped or navicular cells may be present (Figure 11-5). The smear in pregnancy may occasionally contain decidualized stromal cells that have bland nuclei and should not be mistaken for neoplasia or repair. In general, however, pregnancy does not affect the cytologic abnormalities; an abnormal cytosmear has the same significance whether or not a patient is pregnant.

COLPOSCOPY IN THE PREGNANT PATIENT

The colposcopic examination during pregnancy may be very difficult. Adequate visualization is mandatory and usually the largest speculum the patient can accomodate is necessary to retract the prolapsing vaginal walls. The lateral vaginal walls may have to be retracted using either lateral vaginal wall retractors or a condom whose end tip has been removed and rolled onto the speculum. Five percent acetic acid may have to be used, rather than 3%, in order to dissolve the tenacious cervical mucus that may obscure the colposcopic findings (*see* Figure 11-3).

Any atypicality seen at colposcopy during pregnancy may be overinterpreted because of the increased vascularity, and the lesions may be placed into a higher grade because of the angioarchitecture of pregnancy (Figure 11-6, Figure 11-7). As a general rule, it is easier to see the transformation zone (TZ) and the upper extent of an abnormality because of the eversion noted above. The edema and cyanosis also may change the coloration of the lesion: the intensity of whiteness may be somewhat less in contrast to the surrounding tissue. Decidual changes, which can produce both polyplike extru-

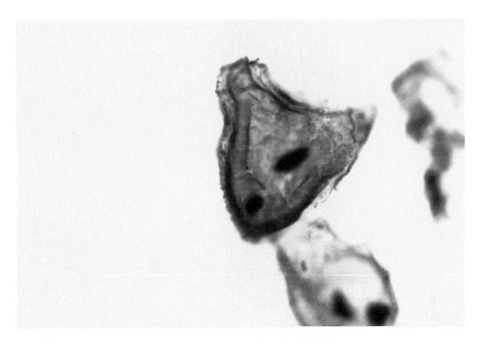

Figure 11-5. Cytosmear from pregnant patient. Note the characteristic navicular, or boat-shaped, cell.

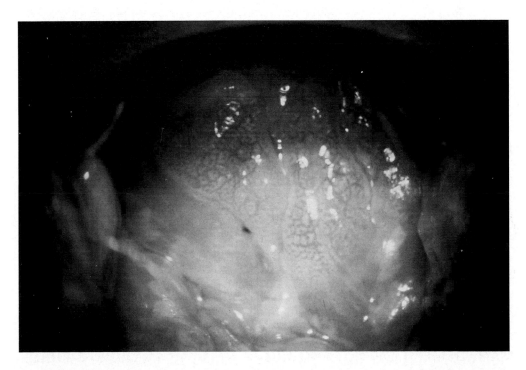

Figure 11-6. Anterior lip of cervix in pregnancy, showing mosaic structure suggestive of CIN. Biopsy revealed decidualization of stroma.

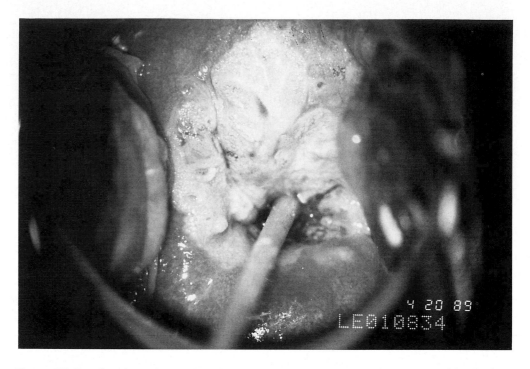

Figure 11–7. Cervix at 25 weeks of gestation with a large, raised, aceto-white lesion with asperities and sharp border. Colposcopy suggests CIN II to III; on biopsy only CIN I with condyloma was present.

sions and the suggestion of a mosaic pattern, may mimic the appearance of invasive cervical cancer. During the process of metaplasia, the newly formed squamous epithelium may exhibit an aceto-white punctation, or mosaic pattern. Despite all of these physiologic changes, atypical blood vessels, the criterion for the diagnosis of frank invasive or microinvasive squamous cell carcinoma, is not one of the changes associated with pregnancy (Figure 11–8a, 11–8b, 11–8c, 11–8d). The presence of this type of atypicality should alert the colposcopist to the possibility of severe disease. Thus, in most patient series of colposcopy performed during pregnancy, severe intraepithelial neoplasia, microinvasive disease, and invasive disease have not been missed.

BIOPSY

Biopsying the cervix during pregnancy can be quite hazardous because the marked increase in vascularity may make bleeding difficult to control. Except in the first trimester of pregnancy, therefore, biopsies of the pregnant cervix should generally be done in an environment in which ancillary equipment (intravenous set-up, local anesthetic, suture material) is available. As a general rule, firm pressure and the use of Monsel's solution (ferric subsulfate) are usually adequate for the control of bleeding. Because of the risk of rupturing the membranes, endocervical curettage is contraindicated during pregnancy. In addition, when taking a Pap smear during pregnancy, the cytobrush should not be used; a wet cotton-tipped applicator should be substituted to sample the endocervical canal.

MANAGEMENT OF THE ABNORMAL CYTOSMEAR DURING PREGNANCY

Abnormal cytology requiring investigation is not uncommon during pregnancy. In the past, evaluation of the abnormal cervix in pregnancy was by cold knife cone biopsy,

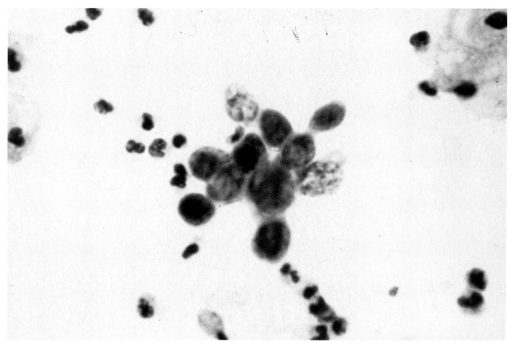

A

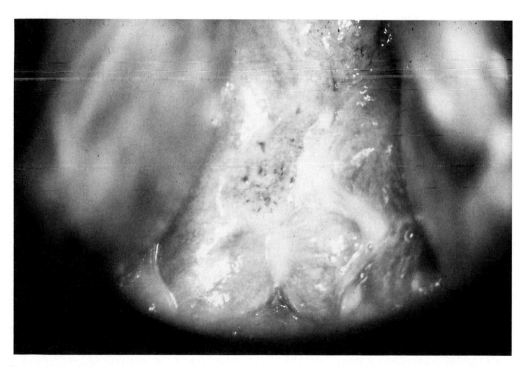

B

Figure 11-8.   A. Atypical cytosmear at 36 weeks of gestation. The nuclei are hyperchromatic, enlarged, and have virtually no cytoplasm. Cytodiagnosis is CIN III. **B.** Cervix at 36 weeks' gestation (*see* Figure 11-8A) prior to acetic acid. Note the group of atypical blood vessels at 9 o'clock. Note how the side walls of the vagina bulge inward. (*Figure continues.*)

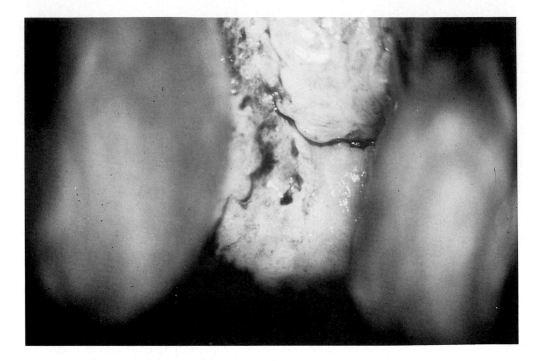

C

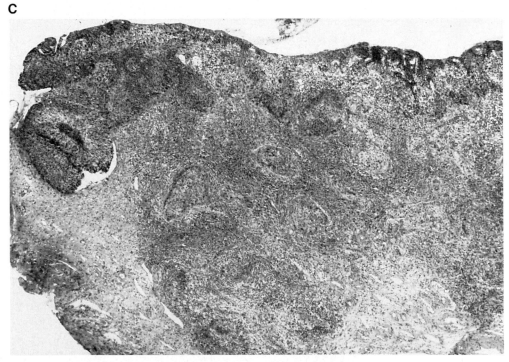

D

Figure 11–8 (continued). C. Cervix after application of acetic acid (*see* Figure 11–8B). Note the intense aceto-white change and friability of the abnormal vessels. **D.** Biopsy of the cervix in the region of the atypical blood vessels, revealing invasive squamous cell cancer. Biopsy at 6 o'clock revealed CIN III. The patient had a cesarian radical hysterectomy and did well.

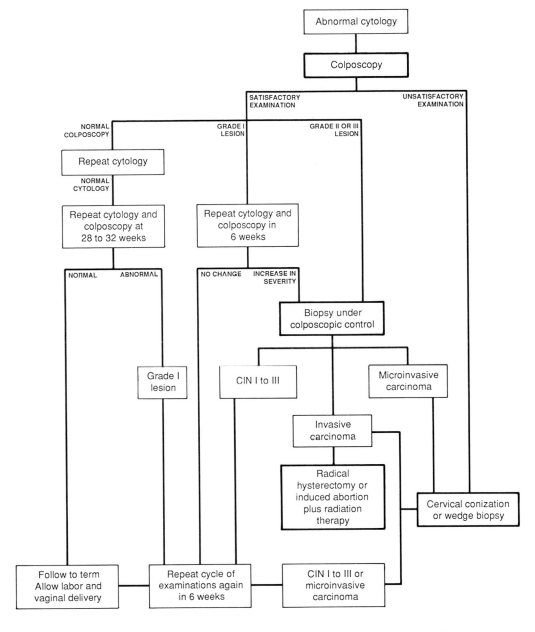

Figure 11-9. Allogram of the management of the atypical cytosmear during pregnancy. *(Reprinted with permission from* Obstetrical Decision Making *by EA Friedman.)*

which posed significant risk to the mother and fetus. A complication rate of 20% to 30% is the acknowledged risk of this procedure during pregnancy. Not only are hemorrhage, premature delivery, and abortion possible, but also inadequacy of the cone biopsy with residual disease occurs in a high proportion of cases.

Colposcopy, however, with directed biopsy obviates the need for conization in 85% to 90% of the patients with abnormal cytology during pregnancy. With the use of the directed colposcopic biopsy, the likelihood of missing an invasive carcinoma of the cervix has virtually been eliminated. In assessing cervical abnormalities during pregnancy certain precautions must be observed:

1. Avoid injury to the fetus.
2. Assessment must take into account alterations of cervical structure and histology secondary to the hormonal and vascular changes of pregnancy as noted previously.
3. The marked edema and vascularity of the pelvic structures, including the cervix, pose the risk of hemorrhage with tissue sampling as already noted.
4. The increased vaginal discharge and bleeding makes colposcopic evaluation more difficult.

Many series have shown that, with expert cytology and colposcopy, biopsy need not be done unless there is a suggestion of microinvasive or invasive disease. Thus, only grade III lesions or those containing atypical blood vessels will be sampled.

When monitoring the patient with an abnormal cytosmear, close surveillence is mandatory. The patients are seen at 6 to 8 week intervals and cytology and colposcopy are performed at each visit. Biopsy, however, is done only if the cytology or colposcopy changes, and the criteria described above are met. The patient is seen 6 to 8 weeks postpartum, at which time she is revaluated with cytology, colposcopy, and directed biopsy. Figure 11–9 outlines a suggested schema for following the abnormal Pap smear during pregnancy.

Chapter 12 | Colposcopy of the Diethylstilbestrol Exposed Female

Diethylstilbestrol (DES), a nonsteroidal estrogen synthesized by Sir Charles Dodd in 1938, was introduced into the United States in the 1940s. It was used primarily for the prevention of miscarriage and other complications of pregnancy. In the 1950s questions were raised about its efficacy; however, it was not until 1971 that the ill effects of its use were delineated. In that year, Herbst and associates reported the development of clear cell adenocarcinoma of the lower genital tract in young women with exposure to DES in utero. Many studies since then have elucidated the various problems associated with such an exposure.

STRUCTURAL CHANGES RESULTING FROM DIETHYLSTILBESTROL EXPOSURE

Embryology

To understand the effects of DES on the lower genital tract requires review of the embryology of this area. As noted in Chapter 3, the stratified squamous epithelium of the vagina and outer cervix is derived from the upward replacement of the original mullerian duct columnar epithelium by squamous cells originating in the urogenital sinus. In utero, DES affects the cervical and vaginal stroma, which, in turn, may cause structural alterations and also interfere with replacement of mullerian duct epithelium. Persistence of the mullerian duct epithelium in the vagina after birth has been termed "adenosis," whereas columnar epithelium on the portio of the cervix has been called "ectopy" or "ectropion."

Ectopy

Table 12–1 summarizes the usual abnormalities associated with in utero exposure to DES. The non-neoplastic gross alterations of the cervix fall into two general categories. The first is ectopy, formerly known as congenital erosion or erythroplakia. At colposcopy, prior to the application of acetic acid, the cervix is red because of the numerous, normal appearing blood vessels in the stroma of the papillae, which are lined by a single layer of columnar epithelium (Figure 12–1, Color Plate 27). After the application of acetic acid, the area noted to be involved is formed of numerous villi (grapes) of columnar epithelium similar to those seen in the native columnar epithelium of the endocervix (Figure 12–2). Occasionally, these grapes may be unusually large, in which case exposure

TABLE 12-1. ABNORMALITIES ASSOCIATED WITH DES EXPOSURE IN UTERO

Female	Male
Non-Neoplastic Changes	**Non-Neoplastic Changes**
Columnar epithelium, portio of cervix (ectopy, erythroplakia)	Epididymal cysts
	Hypotrophic testes
Cervical-vaginal hood (CVH)	Testicular capsular induration
Vaginal membranes and septa	Abnormal semen analysis
Epithelial changes—adenosis	**Neoplastic Changes**
Uterine abnormalities	Not known
Neoplastic Changes	
Clear cell adenocarcinoma	
?Transformation to squamous neoplasia	

to DES should be particularly suspected. Invariably, these patients have other stigmata of in utero DES exposure (Figure 12–3).

As might be anticipated, examination of biopsy specimens from areas of ectopy will demonstrate endocervical type epithelium on the surface and invaginations of the cervix. The luminal surface may be flat or papillary (Figure 12–4). As the DES cohort ages, the columnar epithelium is increasingly replaced by squamous metaplasia (*see below*). Since ectopy is not uncommon in unexposed women, biopsy of the ectocervix is not useful as an aid in establishing the presence of a putative DES related lesion.

Cervical-vaginal Hood

The second gross alteration of the cervix is the so-called cervical-vaginal hood (CVH). This consists of a partial or complete ring or collar of mucosa and stroma at the periphery of the portio (Figure 12–5). In addition, the cervical portio may, on occasion, be ex-

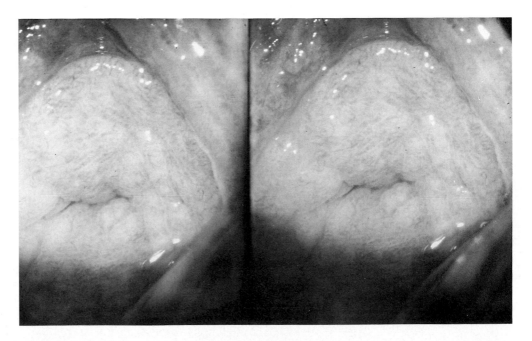

Figure 12-1.   Cervix prior to the application of acetic acid. Portio of the cervix is covered with columnar epithelium containing numerous blood vessels giving the cervix a red color.

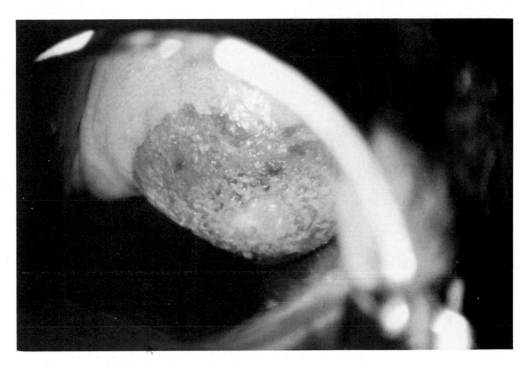

Figure 12–2.   Portio of the cervix after acetic acid. Note that the portio is almost completely covered with columnar epithelium.

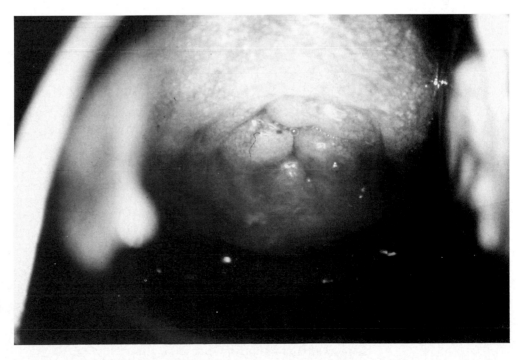

Figure 12–3.   DES cervix. Note the unusually large papillae of columnar epithelium.

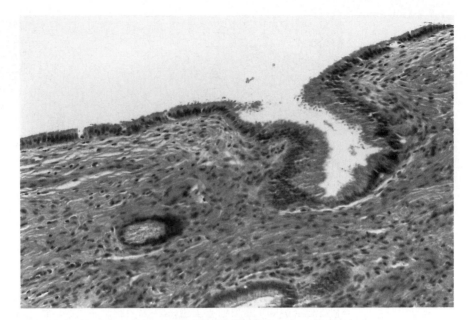

Figure 12–4. Example of cervical ectopy. In this patient, the portio of the cervix was lined by endocervical-type epithelium. Note the presence of endocervical invaginations within the stroma.

tremely small so that it appears to be a "pseudopolyp" in the center of a thick collar (Figure 12–6). The hood often is smoothed out and disappears if the portio is pulled down with a tenaculum or is displaced with the speculum. On the anterior lip of the cervix, the hood often assumes a peaked appearance, the so-called "coxcomb" (Figure 12–7). This group of lesions has no major clinical significance other than as markers of in utero DES exposure.

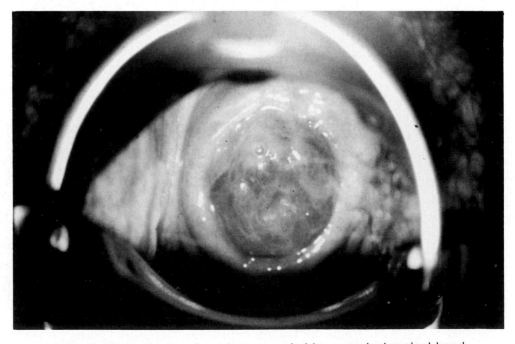

Figure 12–5. Portio of cervix surrounded by a cervical-vaginal hood.

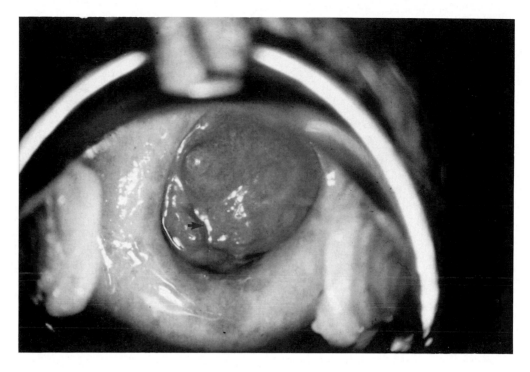

Figure 12-6. Cervix with small portio surrounded by a wide hood producing a pseudopolyp effect. Arrow points to os.

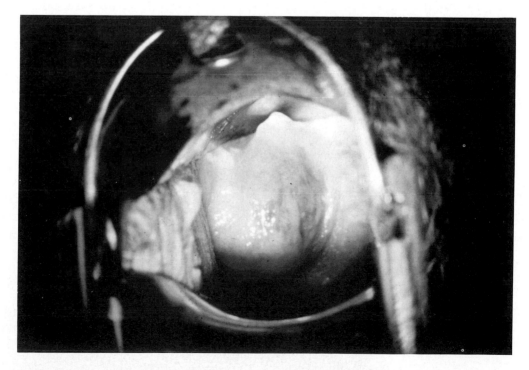

Figure 12-7. Colpophotograph of cervix with peaked appearance of the anterior portion of the hood producing a coxcomb effect. *(Reprinted with permission from* Curr Prob Obstet Gynecol *by L Burke.)*

OTHER VAGINAL CHANGES

In utero exposure to DES may be associated with structural changes in the upper vagina. Vaginal membranes and septa, which are protruding partial or circumferential bands in the upper vagina, may obscure the cervix (Figure 12–8). Since vaginal bands, which occur in about 2% of the exposed females, may result in dyspareunia and may prevent the thorough assessment of the upper one third of the vagina and cervix, they may have to be surgically divided (Figure 12–9). Overall, structural abnormalities of the cervix and vagina have been reported in 22% to 58% of DES exposed women, depending on the nature of the study group (ie, record review versus referral).

Adenosis

Adenosis most often consists of columnar epithelium on the vaginal surface and glands in the underlying stroma; less often, either the surface or the stroma alone is involved. The epithelium may recapitulate all portions of the mullerian system. Although endocervical type columnar cells are most commonly present, about 25% of women will have endometrial-tubal type epithelium within glands (Figure 12–10). Biopsy specimens of adenosis are histologically indistinguishable from those of normal endocervix and can be diagnosed properly only if the pathologist is informed as to the site of origin of the tissue. Over time, adenosis undergoes physiologic squamous metaplasia, with appearances and by mechanisms identical to those of metaplasia in the normal transformation zone (TZ) (*see* Chapter 2) (Figure 12–11). Ultimately, adenosis may be replaced by normal, mature squamous epithelium, although in some women, glands in the stroma may persist unchanged indefinitely.

Based on its natural history, adenosis will vary in appearance when viewed colposcopically. After the application of acetic acid to the cervix and vagina, the most common change is development of an aceto-white epithelium, which is usually sharply delineated on the vaginal wall (Figure 12–12). Most of the aceto-white epithelium in-

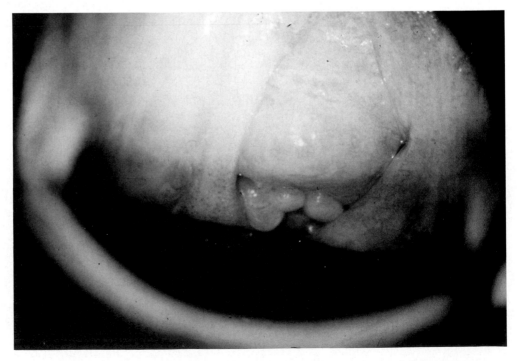

Figure 12-8.   Lateral forniceal folds obscuring portions of the cervix.

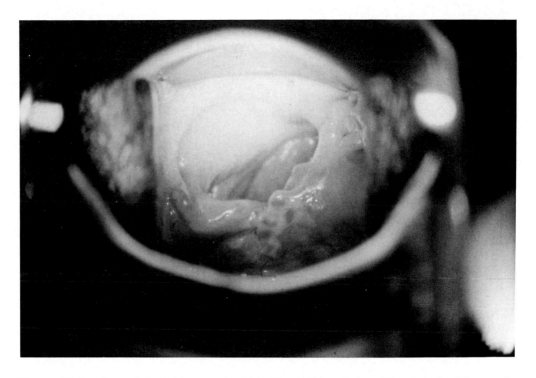

Figure 12-9.   Complete fold around midportion of the vagina. *(Reprinted with permission from* Colposcopy in Clinical Practice *by L Burke and B Mathews.)*

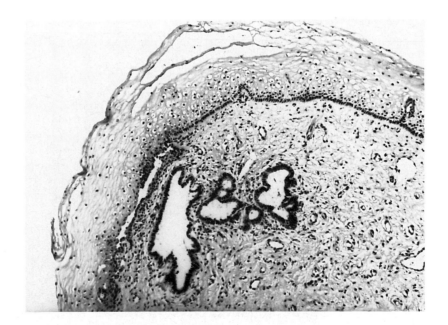

Figure 12-10.   Biopsy of vagina with glands of adenosis in stroma.

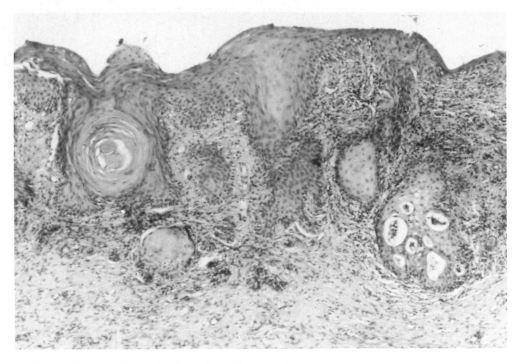

Figure 12–11.   Vaginal adenosis with virtually complete squamous metaplasia.

volves the lateral fornices and anterior vagina, frequently in a triangular pattern that extends cephalad. It frequently involves the posterior fornix as well. In addition, the aceto-white epithelium may have a distinct punctation effect within it (Figure 12–13). Less common is the development of a mosaic pattern, in the same distribution as the aceto-white epithelium (Figure 12–14). Both the aceto-white epithelium and the mosaic structure, correlate with the presence of squamous metaplasia within adenosis. Isolated,

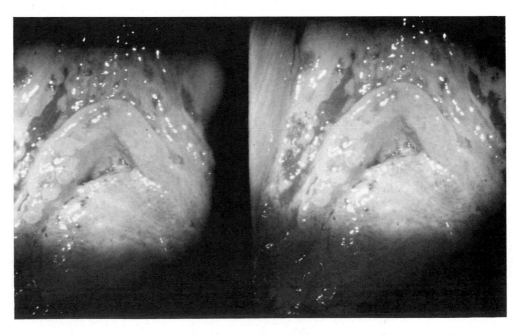

Figure 12–12.   Colpophotograph of adenosis with aceto-white epithelium.

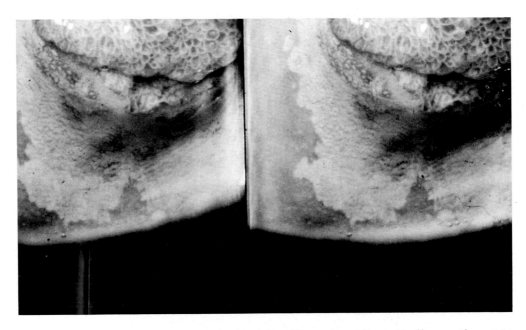

Figure 12–13. Colpophotograph of adenosis with aceto-white epithelium and punctation. *(Reprinted with permission from* Colposcopy in Clinical Practice *by L Burke and B Mathews.)*

irregular areas of columnar epithelium, whose "grapelike" appearance is similar to that seen in ectopy, may also be encountered (Figure 12–15). This finding, which correlates with adenosis having no or minimal squamous metaplasia, is most frequently seen in the very young, DES exposed individual. It is less common today as the exposed cohort has become older. This type of epithelium is most often located in the posterior or lateral fornices high in the vagina.

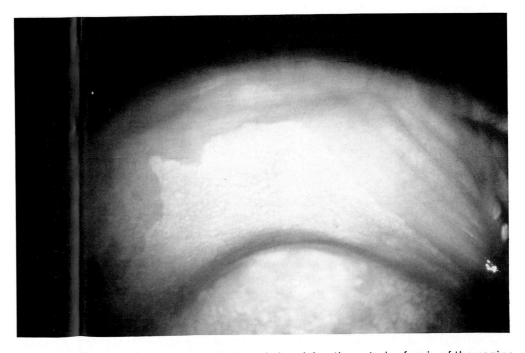

Figure 12–14. Colpophotograph of adenosis involving the anterior fornix of the vagina in a mosaic pattern.

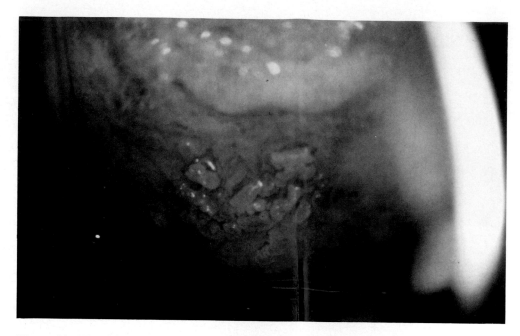

Figure 12–15. Colpophotograph of adenosis with columnar epithelium in the posterior fornix of the vagina.

THE TRANSFORMATION ZONE

Because of the presence of ectopy and adenosis, the TZ in the DES exposed woman is much more extensive than in unexposed females. It may reach the fornices or sidewalls of the vagina in about 80% of these women. The TZ is similar in appearance in both groups of women, however, with islands of columnar epithelium, gland openings, and Nabothian cysts. As already noted, adenosis is characterized colposcopically by a multiplicity of appearances. The most common presentation is aceto-white epithelium alone; mosaic structure is second in frequency, followed by a combination of aceto-white epithelium and mosaic pattern in different areas of the vagina and hood. These three patterns occur in the hood or vagina of almost two thirds of DES exposed patients. Columnar epithelium alone is quite rare, being present in less than 5% of patients.

Cytologically and histologically, tissue from these areas will reflect the degree of metaplasia that is present (Figure 12–16, Figure 12–17). The cytologic positivity of the smears for adenoses will decrease as the patient becomes older and as the metaplastic process becomes mature and is replaced by normal, glycogenated stratified squamous epithelium.

Although high-grade aceto-white and mosaic areas on the cervix in nonexposed women will often demonstrate cervical intraepithelial neoplasia when biopsied, similar degrees of colposcopic abnormalities in the vagina of DES exposed females will usually correlate with immature squamous metaplasia in tissue samples. When these abnormal colposcopic lesions in DES women are studied carefully, the vasculature of the punctation or mosaic, which at first may be suggestive of a severe lesion, has intercapillary distances that are within normal limits and the vessels themselves are fine rather than coarse. These findings are similar to those of immature squamous metaplasia as described in Chapter 3.

Ectopy, the CVH, and adenosis are dynamic lesions, capable of extensive change that becomes more evident with prolonged periods of follow-up observation. Analysis of our follow-up data has shown that of DES exposed women followed for 3 years or longer, ectopy decreased in amount in 75%, with complete disappearance in 30% of

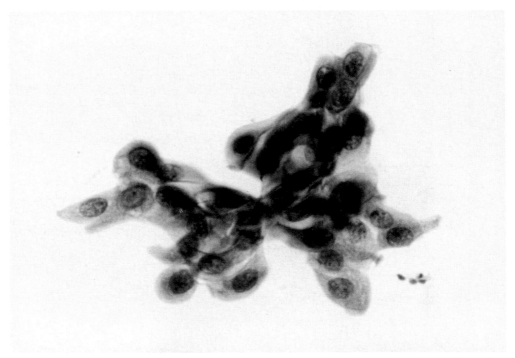

Figure 12-16. Cytosmear from anterior fornix showing squamous metaplastic cells.

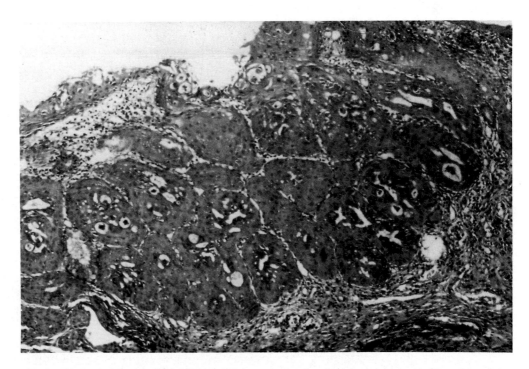

Figure 12-17. Biopsy from the patient in Figure 12-12, demonstrating extensive squamous metaplasia of adenosis.

this group (Figure 12–18a, 12–18b, 12–19a, 12–19b). Resolution was by means of squamous metaplasia. During the same follow-up interval (3 or more years), women with CVH also demonstrated an involution of this lesion. There was complete disappearance of the hood in 45% of patients (Figure 12–20a, Figure 12–20b). The precise mechanisms causing this devolution are unclear, but squamous metaplasia of the surface epithelium and remodeling of the underlying stroma have been implicated. Regardless of the mechanisms, the end result of changes in ectopy and CVH is frequently a smooth contoured cervical portio with a metaplastic TZ, in essence, a cervix that is indistinguishable from the cervix of nonDES exposed women.

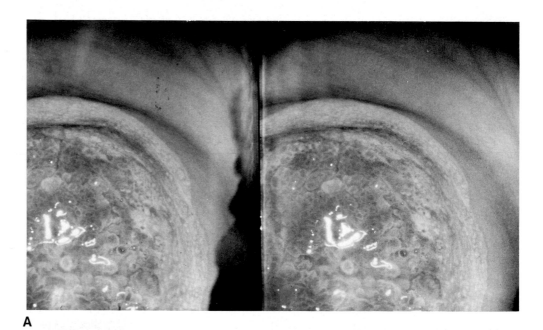

A

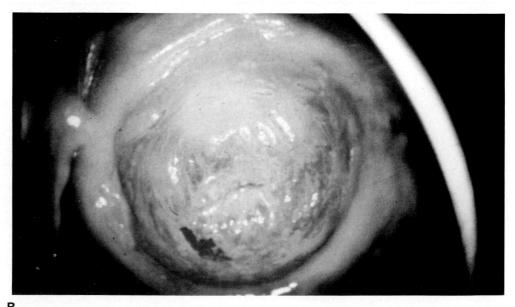

B

Figure 12–18.   A. Cervix with 100% ectopy related to DES exposure. **B.** Cervix of Figure 12–18A showing decrease of ectopy over time. *(Reprinted with permission from* Am J Obstet Gynecol *by D Antonioli et al.)*

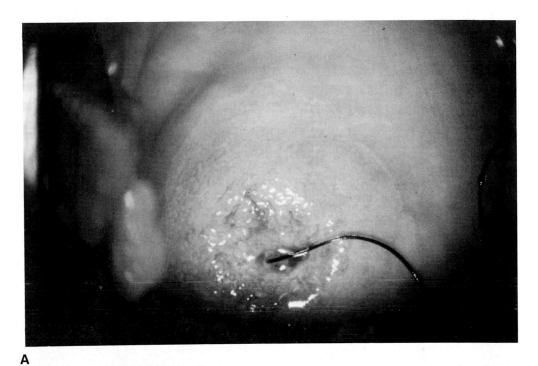

A

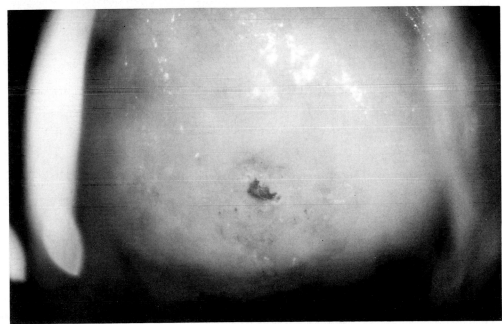

B

Figure 12-19.   A. Cervix with ectopy due to DES exposure. **B.** Cervix of Figure 12-19A showing complete disappearance of the ectopy over time.

Since squamous metaplasia is progressive in the widened TZ represented by ectopy and adenosis, the colposcopic appearance of these lesions also changes over time. Columnar epithelium is the most unstable pattern, decreasing or disappearing by conversion to aceto-white epithelium or mosaic structure in about 60% of women after 3 or more years of observation (Figure 12-21a, 12-21b). Mosaic pattern changes in approximately 30% of the DES cohort, converting to aceto-white or normal mucosa. In addition to being the most common colposcopic appearance in adenosis, aceto-white epithelium (representing advanced squamous metaplasia) is the most stable, changing in less than 20% of women over time. When change does occur in aceto-white epithelium, however, it is chiefly to a normal appearance representing the development of a mature squamous mucosa.

Over time, a significant percentage of the DES cohort will lose lower genital tract stigmata suggestive of in utero exposure to this drug. Therefore, without these stigmata,

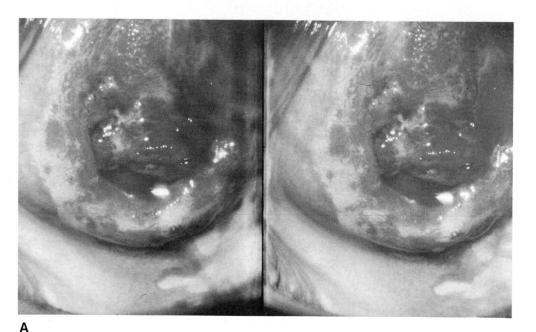

A

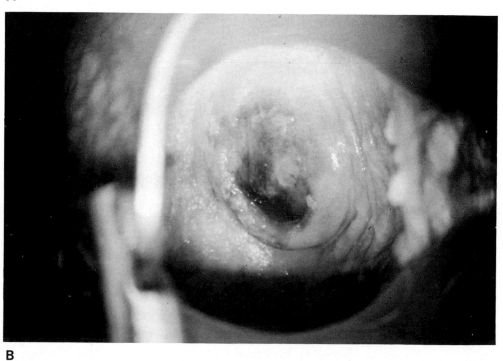

B

Figure 12-20.   A. Cervix with complete CVH associated with DES exposure. **B.** Cervix of Figure 12-20A showing disappearance of the CVH over time. *(Reprinted with permission from* Obstet Gynecol *by L Burke et al.)*

the history of DES exposure will become increasingly important in defining the population at risk for the development of any new lesions with advancing age.

CLEAR CELL ADENOCARCINOMA

The most serious result of in utero exposure to DES has been the development of clear cell adenocarcinoma in young females. The risk of DES daughters developing this

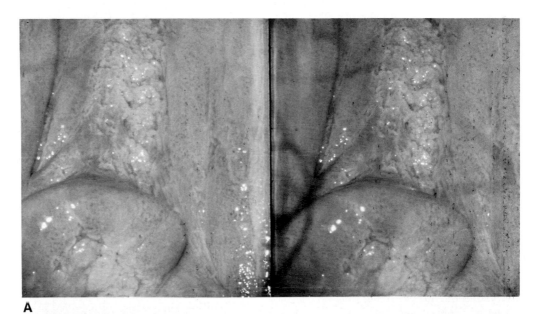

A

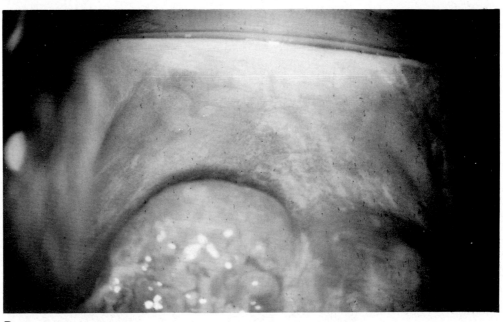

B

Figure 12-21. A. Anterior fornix of vagina in DES exposed female with columnar epithelium. **B.** Anterior fornix of Figure 12–21A 3 years later. The columnar epithelium has been replaced by aceto-white epithelium. Biopsy revealed extensive squamous metaplasia of adenosis. *(Reprinted with permission from* Obstet Gynecol *by L Burke et al.)*

malignancy is approximately 1.4 per 1000 exposed females. These cancers have developed in women aged 7 to 34 years; however, over 90% have been between 15 and 28 years of age at the time of diagnosis. The frequency of this disease in the older exposed woman is as yet unknown, but it should be recalled that prior to the DES era, 60% of clear cell carcinomas were reported in women older than 45 years of age.

Most clear cell adenocarcinomas are found in the upper third of the anterior vaginal wall or on the ectocervix (Color Plate 28). The tumors are typically polypoid, but many are relatively flat or ulcerated. Rarely, the tumor may be small and lie in the lamina propria just beneath an intact mucosa. These latter tumors present as an induration or small nodule best appreciated by palpation of the vaginal walls (Color Plate 29).

Histology

Histologically, clear cell adenocarcinoma is characterized by two predominant growth patterns and two cell types. The more common pattern is characterized by tubules and cysts, the latter often containing papillae (Figure 12–22). The tubules, cysts, and papillae are typically lined by hobnail cells. These are cells with apical bulbous nuclei, covered by a thin rim of cytoplasm (Figure 12–23). Occasionally, the cysts may be lined by flattened, innocous appearing tumor cells. The less common pattern is formed of clear cells whose cytoplasm is filled with glycogen. Clear cells usually grow in solid masses, but occasionally line tubules.

Adenosis, particularly of the endometrial-tubal type, is identified adjacent to most vaginal clear cell cancers. In fact, adenosis is considered to be the precursor of the cancers. It undergoes malignant change through the intermediate step of dysplasia.

Colposcopy

Colposcopically, obvious polypoid or ulcerated cancers are easily recognized. Small, flat, or submucosal tumors may be difficult to appreciate. The only clue to the presence of the latter group of tumors is the appearance of atypical blood vessels (*see* Color Plate

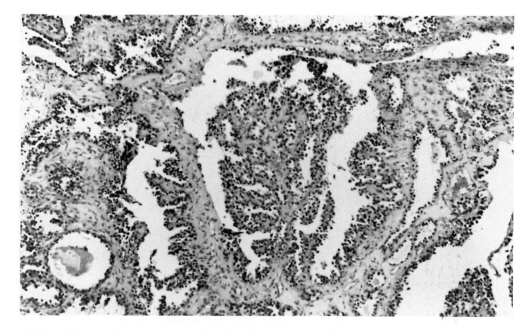

Figure 12–22. Biopsy specimen of clear cell adenocarcinoma showing tubules and papillae. *(Reprinted with permission from* Curr Prob Obstet Gynecol *by L Burke.)*

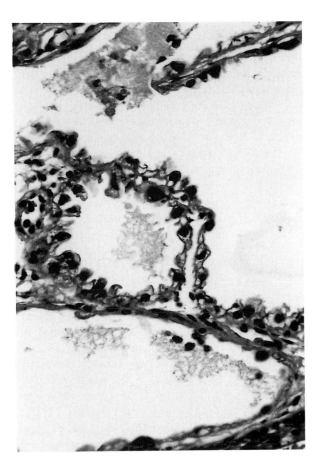

Figure 12-23. Histology of clear cell adenocarcinoma, showing cystic glands lined by cells with hyperchromatic apical nuclei (hobnail cells).

29). The early small lesion close to the surface may produce these atypical blood vessels. In any DES exposed woman, detection of atypical blood vessels should trigger a search for the possibility of an invasive adenocarcinoma.

In addition to local spread, these tumors metastasize by way of the lymphatics and blood vessels. The pelvis is the most common site of tumor recurrence, but there is also a high incidence of pulmonary and clinically apparent supraclavicular lymph node metastases. The treatment of this cancer is primarily surgical and radical, although radiation therapy has been utilized. The actuarial 5-year survival rate is 80%.

CERVICAL NEOPLASIA

Because of the extensive squamous metaplasia found in association with in utero exposure to DES, concern has been raised that dysplasia will occur with greater frequency in these areas of metaplasia. Initial studies did not support this view but Noller and associate's report from the DESAD project has suggested that cervical intraepithelial neoplasia (CIN) is substantially higher in the exposed woman than in controls (15.7 cases compared to 7.9 cases per 1000 persons per year of follow-up). Because of methodologic questions concerning this DESAD study, the relationship between DES exposure and increased risk of subsequently developing squamous cell neoplasia is not considered proven, and further studies are needed. At the present time, vaginal intraepithelial neoplasia (VaIN) has been reported in very few DES exposed women; much longer follow-up is required to determine if the prevalence of VaIN is the same as or greater than in controls.

COLPOSCOPY

Colposcopic evaluation of women exposed to DES has demonstrated the ability of this technique to define the type, frequency, location, and extent of structural and mucosal changes in the cervix and vagina in this population. The advantages of colposcopy in evaluation of these women are similar to those for the evaluation of cervicovaginal lesions in controls. By means of colposcopically directed biopsy, it is possible to sample the most suspicious area for histologic examination; therefore, a large number of blind biopsies from iodine-negative areas in the vagina or cervix are unnecessary. The colposcopic examination, especially of the vagina, does require expertise, because the interpretation of colposcopic changes in DES women is often more difficult than in normal subjects. As already mentioned in the discussion of dysplastic changes, many vaginal grade I and II mosaic and punctation patterns that would be considered suspicious or diagnostic of intraepithelial neoplasia if found in unexposed patients, correlate only with areas of squamous metaplasia in the DES exposed women. Grade III changes, however, invariably signify neoplasia and are predictive of abnormal epithelial changes on biopsy.

Use of the colposcope combined with colpophotographs is uniquely suitable for both the initial evaluation and subsequent follow-up of DES exposed women. Colposcopically abnormal areas that remain unchanged when compared with earlier colpophotographs need not be rebiopsied. In contrast, iodine staining results are nonspecific (Color Plate 30). Nonstaining areas may have to be biopsied repeatedly at follow-up examinations since gross examination gives no information about the nature or stability of the lesion in the unstained area. Although colposcopy cannot definitely diagnose clear cell carcinoma without biopsies, it can detect subtle changes of malignancy (atypical blood vessels, coarse punctation, etc) and thus guide the taking of appropriate biopsies. It is also helpful in delineating the extent of involvement by carcinoma.

INITIAL EXAMINATION

The mere history of in utero exposure to DES should not be an excuse to examine the premenarchal female unless there is a history of bleeding. In general, the initial examination is done at the onset of menarche or by age 14. If the patient is menstruating, she is instructed in the use of tampons; the initial examination is delayed for 6 months. This will allow the pelvic examination to be done using just topical anesthesia applied to the hymeneal ring. If, however, this cannot be accomplished, the initial examination is done under light general anesthesia. A Pedersen virginal speculum will usually allow adequate visualization of the cervix and vaginal canal. Cytology, not only of the cervix and endocervix, but also scrapings from the four vaginal fornices are obtained. All areas of atypical epithelium are photographed and noted. If colposcopy is not available, the cervix and vagina are painted with half-strength Lugol's iodine solution. All areas of colposcopic atypia or noniodine staining should be sampled. Bimanual examination is done in the usual manner. The examination is finished by palpating all four vaginal walls from the fornices to the hymeneal ring. Clear cell adenocarcinoma may first manifest itself as a small nodule just underneath the normal appearing epithelium.

Assuming the cytology is negative and the biopsies only reveal benign adenosis or metaplasia, follow-up examinations are scheduled on a yearly basis. The examination is the same as noted above, except that biopsies are not repeated unless the colposcopy or cytology suggests the development of some form of neoplasia.

Chapter 13 | Common Errors of Cytology and Colposcopy

As noted in Chapter 6, the most important tools for diagnosing and evaluating cervical intraepithelial neoplasia (CIN) are cytology and colposcopy with directed biopsy. The former is a cellular screening technique suggesting that an abnormality exists, whereas the latter, when combined with directed biopsies, may be used to determine the location, type, and severity of the lesion. The combined use of these techniques gives a detection rate of 95% to 99% for CIN. Therefore, in any discussion of errors in the diagnosis of CIN, possible errors in cytology, colposcopy, pathology, or all three must be considered.

CYTOLOGY

Although cervical cytology has been the basic screening method for CIN for over four decades, only in the past 10 years has it been recognized that the method carries a significant false-negative rate. In the United States this rate may be as high as 33% to 40%, but more commonly it ranges from 10% to 15%. Errors in cytology may be divided into those resulting from any of the following areas:

1. The method of sampling, including preservation of the samples.
2. Screening errors.
3. Errors in interpretation.

Sampling Errors and Inadequate Smears

Although the majority of false-negative smears appear to be due to a sampling error, little consensus exists as to the definition of an inadequate smear. It seems obvious, however, that smears that are air-dried, inflammatory, bloody, or thick should be considered inadequate for diagnosis (*see below*).

The method by which smears are taken is also important. In the past, some people advocated sampling of the vaginal pool. Many studies, however, have shown that vaginal pool sampling is of little value in the diagnosis of CIN (although this method may slightly improve detection of endometrial lesions). A single sampling of the ectocervical area also is of scant value. Both the endocervical canal and the portio of the cervix must be sampled to obtain an adequate smear. The most controversial aspect concerning the definition of the adequate smear involves the presence or absence of endocervical cells as an indicator that the critical transformation zone (TZ) has been sampled. Most authors believe that the absence of endocervical cells on a cytosmear constitutes a less than adequate specimen; some clinicians will accept the presence of endocervical mucus to be of itself evidence of an adequate smear. The use of newer sampling modalities such as the cervical cytobrush markedly improves the yield of endocervical cells to greater than 95% of cases and decreases the false-negative rate (Figure 13–1).

Another aspect of smear preparation leading to errors in interpretation is contamination of the smear by lubricants (such as Lubafax) from the examiner's glove. Such smears are highly inadequate because cellular detail is obscured by the lubricant (Figure 13–2). Smears that are air-dried will contain cells in which nuclei are blown-up ("ballooned"), an artifact that may lead to an erroneous diagnosis (Figure 13–3). Formalin is not an adequate fixative because it damages or destroys cellular detail (Figure 13–4). Loss of cell detail is a particular problem in evaluating the gray zone of atypia to mild dysplasia. Therefore, a cytosmear must be immediately fixed in 95% alcohol or flooded by spray fixative.

Taking smears during the menses or in the course of an infection may make interpretation difficult because of excessive erythrocytes and inflammatory cells (Figure 13–5). This, however, should not preclude the examiner from taking a smear at the time of menses because many times the smear can be properly evaluated. If the smear is unsatisfactory, the laboratory should report this to the examiner, and a repeat smear can be done. Cytologic interpretation of atypical smears is greatly aided by an adequate clinical history including hormonal status (ie, last menstrual period, pregnancy, postpartum, or menopausal status), prior abnormal smears, surgery, hormonal therapy, and previous radiation or chemotherapy.

Errors in Interpretation

The false-negative diagnostic rate for CIN for single smears when compared to tissue specimens is usually about 25%. Since approximately one third of this false-negative rate may be attributable to interpretive errors that may occur even in the best laboratory,

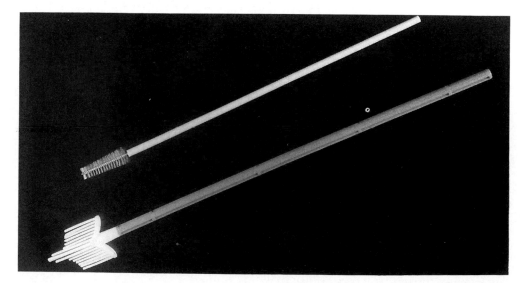

Figure 13-1. "Cytobrush" *(top)* and "Unimar" *(bottom)* plastic cytosmear samplers. Endocervical cell yield is improved using these to sample the endocervical canal.

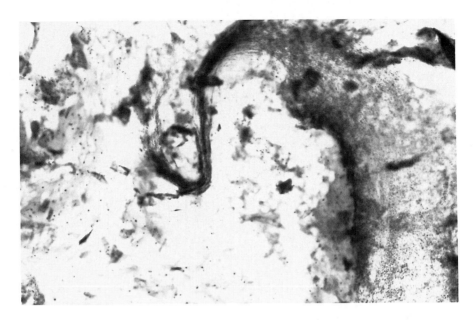

Figure 13-2. Lubricant obscuring the details of a cytosmear.

it is encumbent on the clinician to select a high quality laboratory. Unfortunately, few mechanisms exist for objectively evaluating laboratories. Although laboratories should conform to the standard of rescreening 10% of randomly selected negative cases, this measure might not identify the small number of missed cases and does not address the problem of specificity. The best method for quality control is comparison of cytologic with histologic findings and long-term follow-up. Unfortunately, unless the laboratory is also receiving cervical biopsies, this approach is almost impossible, especially when a large volume of material is being screened. In the absence of identifiable criteria and

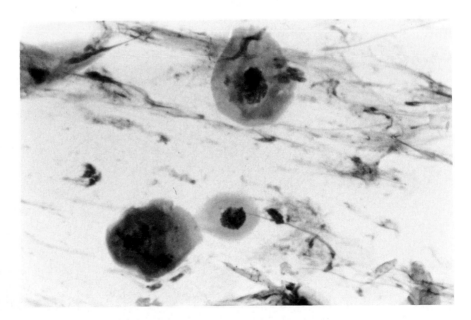

Figure 13-3. Cytologic smear with air drying artifact. Note the poor nuclear detail and "blown up" appearance of the entire cell.

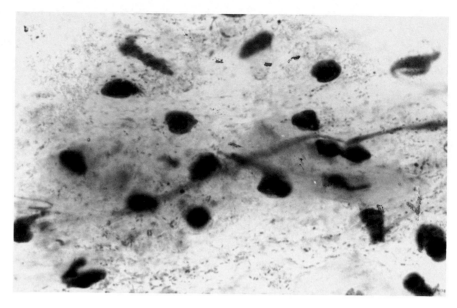

Figure 13–4. Poor preservation of cells secondary to fixation in formalin.

external quality assurance, clinicians may wish to inquire of their cytology laboratories as to the credentials of the medical and technical directors, volume of work per screener, method of quality assurance, and correlations of cytology and tissue in that particular laboratory. New federal regulations for the purpose of cytology quality control include proficiency testing for laboratories. Whether or not these new measures will meet the goal of improving the sensitivity of cytosmears is as yet unknown.

Other Diagnostic Problems

Other problems in the diagnosis of significant CIN include the cytosmear that contains mildly atypical cells and how best to follow patients with such smears (Figure 13–6). Although many recent studies have addressed the sensitivity issue, few have looked at

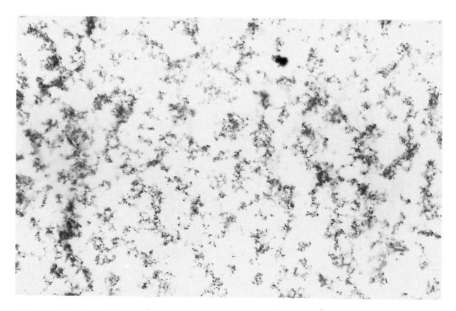

Figure 13–5. Bloody cytosmear. The underlying cellularity is obscured.

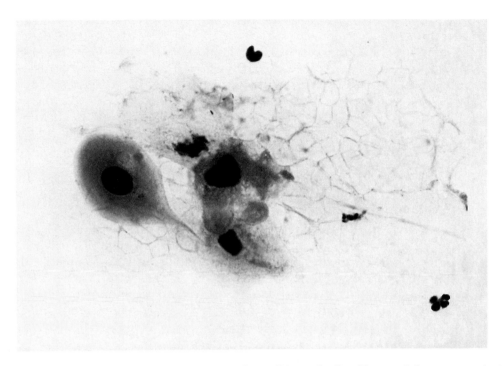

Figure 13-6. Cytologic smear demonstrating mild atypicality. The nuclei are somewhat enlarged in comparison to normal intermediate cells. There are, however, no significant alterations of the chromatin or hyperchromasia.

the false-positives in cytology. In order to increase sensitivity, a laboratory may report more borderline cytosmears as atypical, resulting in a decrease in specificity. It has been shown, however, that if colposcopy is done on patients with the mildly atypical smears, as many as 18% to 25% of them will have significant disease. Since the cytosmear may be negative within 5 years prior to diagnosing invasive carcinoma, all patients who have an abnormal smear indicating the possibility of neoplasia, irrespective of the grade, should be referred for colposcopy on the first abnormal smear. Cytosmears with only mildly dysplastic cells may be obtained from patients with more severe histopathologic lesions; many patients with smears that indicate CIN I to II will have, in fact, CIN III, microinvasive disease, or even invasive disease on further evaluation.

COLPOSCOPIC ERRORS

Errors of colposcopy may result from:

1. Overinterpretation of minor lesions.
2. Pregnancy.
3. Incomplete visualization of the TZ.
4. Errors associated with biopsy technique.
5. The postmenopausal state.

Overinterpretation

The major value of colposcopy has been to discover and separate those patients who have the preclinical phase of disease (CIN) from patients who have invasive carcinoma. Thus, it is imperative that when evaluating the cervix, invasive carcinoma should be ruled out before the decision to do definitive therapy has been made.

One of the most common errors in colposcopy is either overdiagnosing or under-diagnosing the colposcopic image. As a general rule, the clinician is more likely to over-diagnose than underdiagnose a particular lesion. The teaching in colposcopy is that an atypical TZ should be regarded as harboring a neoplastic lesion. By grading the atypical TZ as already described in Chapter 5, the experienced colposcopist is able to correlate the colposcopic image with the histologic diagnosis. Many colposcopists, however, both experienced and neophyte, have been frustrated on biopsying a grade II atypical TZ, anticipating the presence of some form of CIN, only to receive a pathology report with a diagnosis of "squamous metaplasia with acute and chronic cervicitis." The colposcopic lesions that are the source of this discrepancy are usually sharply defined aceto-white areas with a flat surface (*see* Figures 5–23, 5–24, 6–8a, 6–8b, 6–8c). There usually are no visible terminal vessels, and one can see only minimally developed vascular struc-tures. The importance of these lesions is that, in fact, some of them are CIN. The error occurs if they are interpreted only as areas of metaplasia and, therefore, are not biop-sied. As a result, those lesions representing CIN will be missed. This type of lesion is also being seen more frequently now in the form of the flat condyloma, which carries its own set of implications, as already discussed in Chapter 10.

The importance of the various colposcopic images, grade for grade, in terms of signifying the presence of neoplasia may be listed in the following order:

1. Atypical blood vessels (*see* Figures 5–10, 5–22).
2. Aceto-white epithelium (*see* Figures 5–26, 5–27).
3. Mosaic and punctation (*see* Figures 5–2, 5–5, Color Plate 9).
4. Leukoplakia (*see* Figure 5–20).

Atypical blood vessels, the hallmark of microinvasive and invasive disease, are the most important colposcopic images to recognize. Leukoplakia, on the other hand, is usually associated with human papilloma virus (HPV) infection and is much less im-portant unless it is covering an underlying severe CIN. Punctation and mosaic struc-tures, which are both vascular aberrations, are significant only when they are present within a field of aceto-white epithelium. Therefore, aceto-white change is the second most important colposcopic image because it carries not only an intrinsic association with CIN but also provides the background in which vascular changes must be evaluated. Unfortunately, grade I to II punctation and mosaic structures with minimal aceto-white change are visually dramatic, and the neophyte must be alert to the fact that his or her eyes will be drawn to these changes, ignoring a grade II to III aceto-white lesion with-out vascular changes elsewhere. A grade I punctation or mosaic pattern carries with it much less significance than a grade III aceto-white change.

Pregnancy

Errors may occur in association with pregnancy. The physiologic and morphologic changes of pregnancy may alter the character of the cervix to produce an atypical col-poscopic appearance of aceto-white, mosaic, or punctation change, (*see* Chapter 11). It is not unusual to have colposcopic images related to the benign changes of pregnancy that in the nonpregnant cervix would be significant CIN.

Incomplete Visualization

Probably the most important source of error during the colposcopic examination relates to the incomplete visualization of the endocervical canal. Evaluation of the endocervix may be accomplished, as already noted in previous chapters, by the use of cotton-tipped applicators (*see* Figure 2–8), various hooks (*see* Figure 2–9), or endocervical specula (*see* Figure 2–12, Color Plate 14). A newer technique involves using either the contact (Figure 13–7) or the Hamou hysteroscope (Figure 13–8) to evaluate the squamocolumnar junc-tion. These techniques, however, do require special instrumentation and training and, therefore, are not yet applicable to the general practice of gynecology.

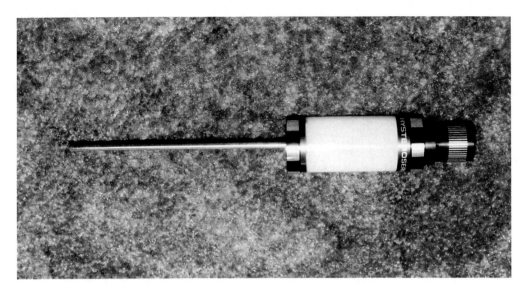

Figure 13-7.   Contact hysteroscope that uses ambient light to visualize the endocervical canal.

Errors in Curettage Technique

The most common method of sampling the endocervical canal is by use of the endocervical curette. Improper technique in using the endocervical curette will lead to an inordinate number of false-positive specimens. The usual techniques of dragging the curette down across the portio of the cervix after the curettage may dislodge strips of cervical

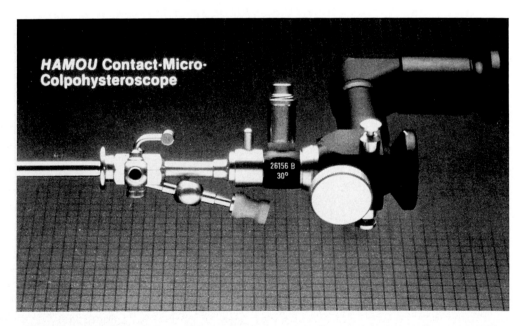

Figure 13-8.   Hamou hysteroscope, used to visualize the endocervix and the endometrial cavity. In the endocervical canal, the visualization is enhanced by staining the cells with Waterman's blue ink.

dysplastic epithelium not attached to stroma (Figure 13–9). It is difficult, if not impossible, for the pathologist to determine the origin of such fragments; hence, the curettage will be diagnosed as positive for dysplasia even though the canal may actually be negative.

The curettage should be performed with the curette remaining within the endocervical canal, then being gently removed; all the material should be collected either on telfa sponges or other appropriate material and placed in fixative. All fragments of tissue and blood should be included in the specimen to achieve maximum diagnostic yield. Following the curettage, colposcopic examination of the cervix should be repeated to ascertain whether or not the portio has been scraped, resulting in potential contamination of the specimen.

Because invasive carcinomas have been missed during colposcopic evaluation, various authors have recommended that all colposcopic evaluations include a routine endocervical curettage (ECC), especially if the patient is to receive conservative therapy for CIN. Obviously, routine ECC should be performed if the colposcopist does not have the experience to readily recognize normal endocervical epithelium or if he or she is not certain of the location of the physiologic squamocolumnar junction and extent of the TZ. If the colposcopist is experienced, however, this particular procedure may be omitted. If the tissue in the ECC is significantly abnormal (namely, CIN II to CIN III or worse) then conization is indicated.

The Postmenopausal State

The postmenopausal state is confusing to the colposcopist for two reasons. First, the squamocolumnar junction is usually within the endocervical canal (*see* Chapter 4) and unavailable for inspection, biopsy, or both. The second problem relates to mucosal atrophy (*see* Chapter 5), in which the vessels are very prominent and may be misinterpreted as being abnormal. Both problems can frequently be helped by "estrogenizing" the patient for 2 or 3 weeks before the examination. It has been shown that unsatisfactory colposcopy can be made satisfactory 40% of the time by the use of 1.25 mgm con-

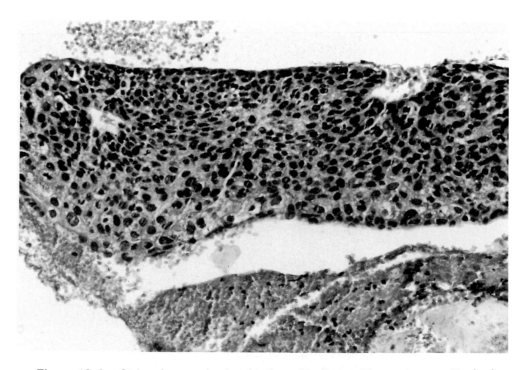

Figure 13–9. Strip of severely dysplastic epithelium with no stroma attached.

jugated estrogen daily for 2 or 3 weeks. This may be given orally or per vaginum in the form of a cream.

Other Possible Errors

Other possible errors during the colposcopic examination are improper biopsy technique, inadequate biopsy of the abnormal TZ, and improper orientation of the specimen (*see* Chapter 2). It is imperative that every colposcopist have a close working relationship with his or her pathologist. Indeed, it is not sufficient for the colposcopist to give the pathologist the small biopsy specimen without reviewing his or her own slides. Conversely, the pathologist should observe colposcopic examinations so that he or she will understand the clinical correlates of the histologic findings and also appreciate the problems in taking biopsies and the reasons the biopsies are necessarily small.

The various instruments for taking biopsies have already been discussed in Chapter 2. The instruments must be sharp, and should cut, rather than squeeze, the tissue when the biopsies are taken. Squeezed biopsy specimens are very difficult for the pathologist to interpret (*see* Figure 2–18, Figure 2–19). Each biopsy specimen should not only be oriented, but should also be labeled so that the colposcopist can compare his or her colposcopic evaluation with the pathologic diagnosis. As already described in Chapter 2, various techniques may be used for keeping the biopsies separate and identified. When the clinical impression and the histologic diagnosis concur, the colposcopist can be certain that conization is unnecessary.

As already noted in Chapter 2, we firmly believe that all biopsies should be taken while looking through the colposcope so that past pointing will not occur and the lesion be missed. We reiterate, however, that if this cannot be done, then the lesion should be marked with Lugol's iodine as described. In addition to biopsying the proper area, it is also imperative that in large lesions, ample sampling be performed rather than simply taking one specimen from the area of greatest abnormality. This is necessary in order to avoid missing any significant pathology.

In summary, among the potential errors of the colposcopic method, incomplete visualization of the TZ is the most important; poor biopsy technique and inadequate biopsy follow close behind. Failure to correlate the biopsy with cytology or poor orientation of the biopsy material also contributes to error in evaluating colposcopic images. Most importantly, the experience of the colposcopist is the major factor in determining the potential for error: the greater the experience, the less likely that error will occur.

Chapter 14 | <u>Cervicography</u>

INTRODUCTION

For the past several decades, the attack on invasive squamous cell carcinoma of the cervix has been dependent on the use of the cervical cytosmear for screening and on colposcopy to determine the extent and severity of the lesion. As a result, the American Cancer Society has reported that the number of new cases of invasive squamous cell carcinoma per year has dropped from 20,000 in 1971 to about 15,000 in 1984. A meteoric rise in the number of cervical intraepithelial neoplasia (CIN) lesions, however, has occurred during this interval; currently, an estimated 45,000 new cases of CIN III and about 200,000 new cases of all grades of CIN are identified in the United States each year.

Since the cervix is one of the most accessible internal organs, theoretically we should be able to prevent the development of invasive squamous cell carcinoma by discovering and eradicating the CIN lesion. Although the combination of cytology and colposcopy has been effective, there are still problems that prevent our attaining the goal of complete eradication of cervical neoplasa.

The high false-negative rate for cytology is one such problem as already discussed in Chapter 13. A second group of problems relates to colposcopy; some of these issues were discussed in Chapter 13. Successful colposcopy depends on the expertise of the examiner. Many factors contribute to developing this expertise, one of which is an adequate number of patients with neoplasia. Equally important is the availability of consultation or supervision of the neophyte colposcopist so that he or she learns to interpret the colposcopic image correctly. Unfortunately, the physician often takes a two to three day postgraduate education course, purchases an expensive colposcope, and, despite all the warnings given in the course, becomes an instant expert and changes his or her method of treating CIN. Conization is abandoned and conservative ablation of the lesion is done without adequately ruling out invasive disease. The two most common errors of colposcopy are:

1. The nonrecognition of unsatisfactory colposcopy where the squamocolumnar junction is not really seen.
2. The nonrecognition of atypical blood vessels compatible with microinvasion or early invasion.

The colposcopic picture of atypical vessels compatible with these lesions is usually much less striking than the pattern of CIN III with coarse punctation, mosaic pattern, or both, or with grade III aceto-white change. It is easy to train gynecologists to recognize CIN, but it is difficult to obtain expertise in the recognition of atypical blood vessels because the general gynecologist may not see even one case of micro- or macroinvasive cervical cancer per year.

In an attempt to resolve these complex problems, a new diagnostic technique called cervicography was developed in 1981 by Adolf Stafl. Among its objectives were the supplementation of cytology in the routine screening of the cervix and the photographic documentation of cervical abnormalities. The latter image could be evaluated by expert colposcopists and thus provide consultation, teaching, and advice for the neophyte.

INSTRUMENTATION

The cervicography instrument consists of a 35mm camera with a 100mm macrolens and 50 mm extension ring. A ring flash unit and intensive light for use in focusing are attached to the front of the lens (Figure 14–1). To achieve constant magnification, the f-stop of the lens is fixed to 0.9 mm. An electronic database is attached to the back of the camera, permitting the dialing of a six digit number that is recorded in the corner of the slide (Figure 14–2). The duration of the flash is 1/2000 of a second and, therefore, the camera can be hand-held; the hand vibrations of the operator will not affect the quality of the picture.

TECHNIQUE

The cervix is visualized with a self-retaining speculum. Excess mucus is removed with a cotton swab and the cervix washed with 4% to 5% acetic acid. The hand-held cerviscope is focused on the cervix by moving the entire system back and forth. When the cervix is in axis with the camera line, acetic acid is reapplied. Two cervigrams are then taken. This can be done by the physician or by a nurse or technician after a short period of training; no expertise in colposcopy is required. The camera does not come in contact with the patient, and no risks to the patient are involved.

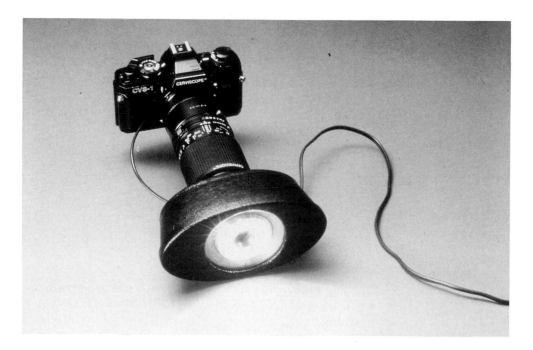

Figure 14–1.   Thirty-five millimeter camera with 100 mm macrolens, 50 mm extension ring, and ring flash unit with intensive light for focusing.

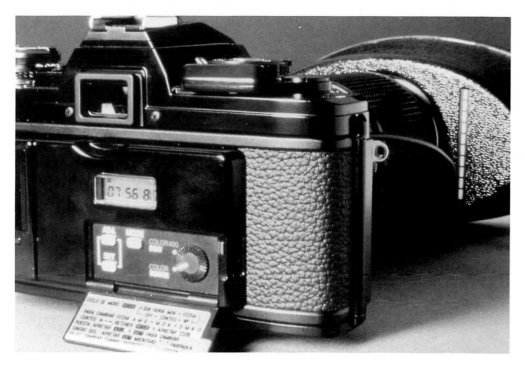

Figure 14-2. Electronic database at back of 35 mm camera.

Optimal photographic results are achieved with the use of Ektochrome or Fujichrome ASA 200 film. The cervigrams will provide a nonmagnified image of the cervix and upper vagina. The depth of field is such that the entire cervix is in view.

The slide is projected onto a plain white (not lenticular) screen, 2 m wide, and the projection observed from a distance of 1 m in a darkened room, using a carousel projector with a stack loader and remote control for focusing. A small penlight aids in recording the findings.

The observed magnification is about the same as that with the colposcope. Table 14-1 demonstrates the method for estimating the magnification on the screen observed from a given distance. The size of the lesion (as well as intercapillary distances) can be determined utilizing the formula in Table 14-2. The apparent magnification on the screen depends on the distance from which the screen is observed. By moving closer to and farther away from the screen it is possible to change magnification, providing an effect similar to changing the magnification on the colposcope.

The cervigrams are sent to a central laboratory for processing (National Testing Laboratories, St Louis) and then forwarded to expert colposcopists, who have undergone training and accreditation by examination in cervicography reporting. The results of the evaluation are then sent back to the individual who took the cervigram (Table 14-3).

TABLE 14-1. MAGNIFICATION ON SCREEN OBSERVED FROM A DISTANCE

$W \times 0.7/3.6 \times 30/D = M$

W = Width of screen in centimeters
D = Distance from screen in centimeters
M = Magnification on screen
Example (screen 150 cm observed from 1 m) $150 \times 0.7/3.6 \times 30/100 = 9.6$

TABLE 14–2. CALCULATION OF SIZE OF LESION

S/M = A
S = Size on screen
M = Magnification (W × 0.7/3.6 = 29.1 for 150 cm screen)
A = Actual size
Example (lesion on screen 12 cm) 12/29.1 − 0.41 cm = 41 mm

REPORTING

The same diagnostic principles apply to cervicography as to colposcopy in interpreting the lesions. Thus, surface contour, sharpness of margin of the lesion, color tone, and vascular patterns are all analyzed (Figures 14–3, 14–4, 14–5, 14–6).

The results of examining the cervigram are reported in one of five categories (Table 14–3). The first category is *negative*. Within this category are cases in which:

1. The squamocolumnar junction and the transformation zone (TZ) are fully visible (Figure 14–7).
2. The squamocolumnar junction is not fully visible but the components of the TZ are visible.
3. The squamocolumnar junction and TZ are not visible but all else is negative (Figure 14–8).

In the latter situation an endocervical smear is essential. A report of negative is followed by the recommendation that a Pap smear and cervigram be repeated in 1 year.

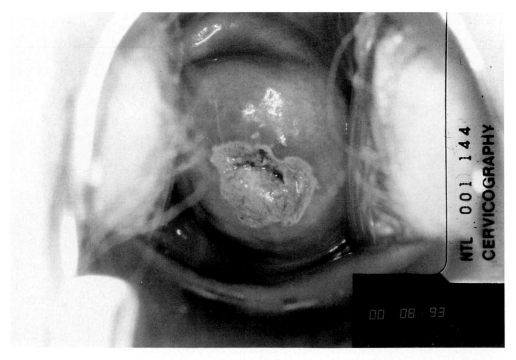

Figure 14–3.   Cervigram of normal transformation zone. Columnar epithelium undergoing squamous metaplasia is evident.

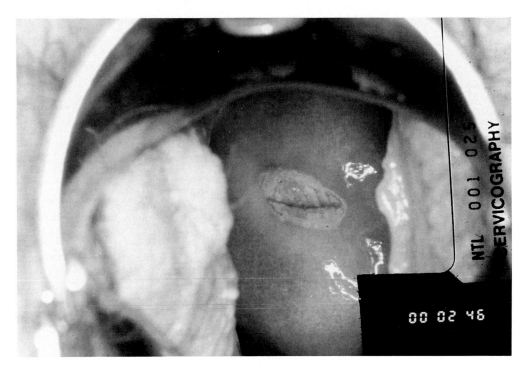

Figure 14-4. Cervigram of a normal TZ.

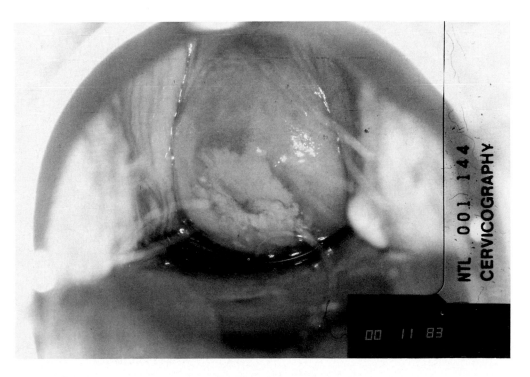

Figure 14-5. Cervigram showing a flat, grade I lesion with feathery borders. Biopsy revealed metaplasia with HPV infection.

TABLE 14-3. EXAMPLE OF CERVIGRAM REPORT FORM

☐ **Negative**—Repeat cervigram and Pap smear annually.

1. _____ Squamocolumnar junction and transformation zone are fully visible.

2. _____ Squamocolumnar junction is not fully visible. Components of the transformation zone are visible.

3. _____ Squamocolumnar junction and transformation zone are not visible. Endocervical smear essential.

☐ **Atypical**—Repeat cervigram and Pap smear in 6 months.

1. _____ Papilloma/condyloma (HPV infection) outside transformation zone.

2. _____ Atypical immature squamous metaplasia.

3. _____ Trivial change of doubtful significance.

☐ **Positive**—Colposcopy recommended.

Lesion morphology: Compatible with:

_____ aceto-white epithelium   1. _____ minor grade lesion (CIN I and II; HPV infection in transformation zone)

_____ punctation

_____ mosaic   2. _____ major grade lesion (CIN III)

_____ atypical vessels   3. _____ invasive cancer

☐ **Technically defective**—Retake cervigram!

1. _____ View of cervix obscured by:

_____ mucus   _____ blood   _____ speculum   _____ vaginal wall

2. _____ Insufficient acetic acid *or* cervigrams taken too late after second application of acetic acid

3. _____ Out of focus

_____ overexposed

_____ underexposed

☐ **Other**—(Vagina, vulva, penis, anus; see comments)

Comments: _____

_____

_____

_____

Evaluated by: _____ Date _____

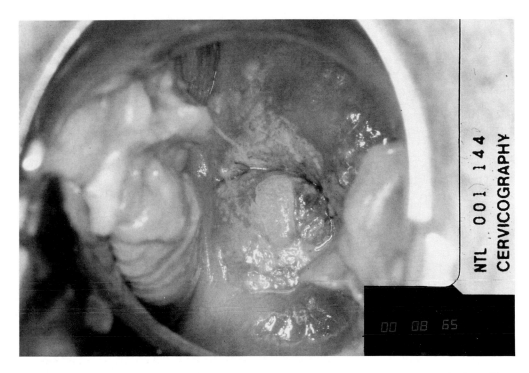

Figure 14-6. Cervigram of an essentially normal TZ, showing at 6 o'clock the effect of metaplasia; the papillae show opacity and whiteness. Biopsy revealed metaplasia.

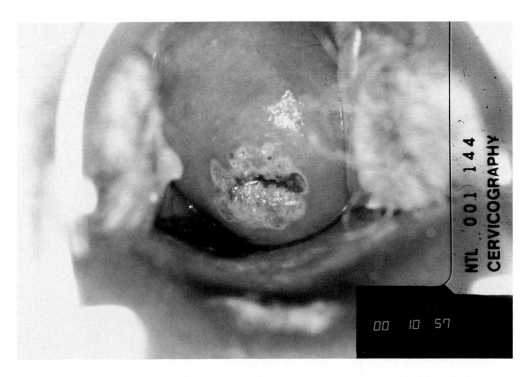

Figure 14-7. Negative cervigram. The squamocolumnar junction and TZ are fully visible.

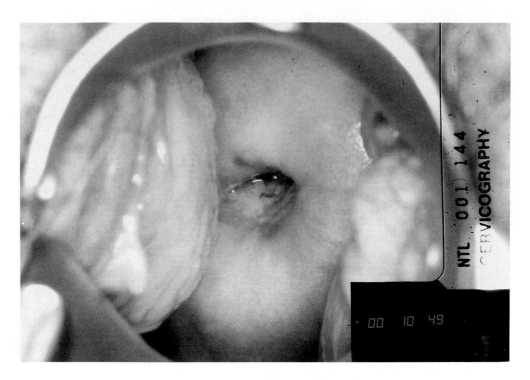

Figure 14–8. Negative cervigram. The squamocolumnar junction is not fully visible, but elements of the TZ are seen.

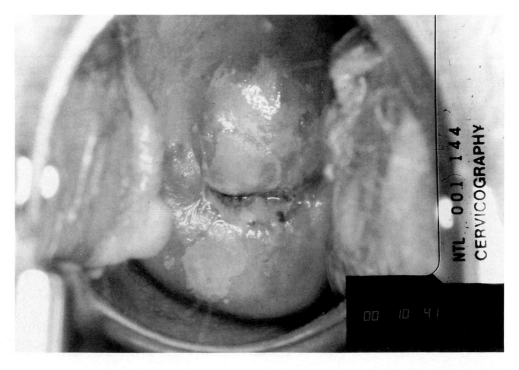

Figure 14–9. Atypical cervigram. Aceto-white lesions on both lips of the cervix. Several lesions are not attached to the squamocolumnar junction. Biopsy revealed condyloma.

The second category is *atypical*. This category includes patients with papilloma/condyloma (human papilloma virus [HPV] infection) outside the TZ, atypical immature metaplasia, and trivial changes of doubtful significance (Figure 14–9, Color Plate 31). A repeat Pap smear and cervigram in 6 months are advised.

The third category is *positive* and requires colposcopic follow-up. Aceto-white epithelium, punctation, mosaic pattern, or atypical blood vessels are present (Figure 14–10, Figure 14–11, Color Plate 32). These findings are compatible with minor grade lesions (CIN I to II, HPV), major grade lesions (CIN III), or invasive cancer.

Technically defective is the fourth category. In this instance the cervigram has to be retaken (Figure 14–12). The deficiency may be due to the cervix being obscured by mucus, blood, the speculum, or the vaginal wall. Also, insufficient acetic acid may have been used or the cervigram taken too late after the second application of the acid. Other causes of defective pictures include out of focus cervigrams and under- or overexposed film.

A final category of *other* is included to describe cervigrams of the vagina, vulva, penis, or anus. These are described in the same fashion as for colposcopy of these areas.

Results

In Stafl's original study, cervicography was performed in 738 women. In 28 women (3.4%) cervicography was technically defective. It was possible to evaluate 700 cervigrams. These were from two groups of patients: (1) 296 patients who had abnormal cytologic findings and were referred to a colposcopic clinic for evaluation. In these patients, the diagnostic accuracy of cervicography in comparison with colposcopy was evaluated. (2) 404 patients who had no previous abnormal cytologic examination; in these patients, screening cervicography was done. Among the 296 patients with correlation of colposcopic and cervicographic findings with biopsy, the differences were not significant, and both methods had comparable diagnostic accuracy. Cervicography was within one histologic degree of accuracy in 93.1% of cases and colposcopy in 92%.

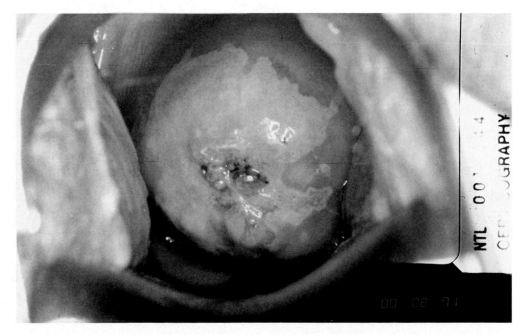

Figure 14–10. Positive cervigram, with wide atypical change consisting of aceto-white epithelium. Biopsy revealed CIN I to II, with condylomatous features.

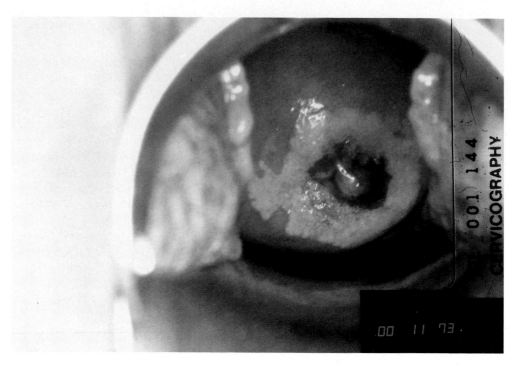

Figure 14-11. Positive cervigram, with circumferential change. Grade I to II mosaic pattern on the posterior cervical lip. Biopsy showed CIN I to II.

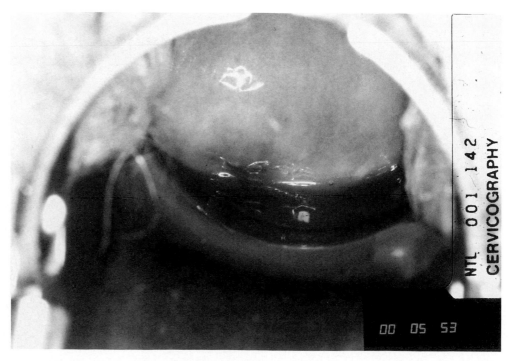

Figure 14-12. Technically defective cervigram. The cervical os is not in axis with the vagina, and therefore, the cervix cannot be evaluated.

Among the 404 patients who had cervicography screening and who had no previous abnormal cytologic screening, cervicography was negative in 239 patients (72.5%), suspicious in 35 patients (8.7%) and unsatisfactory in 76 (18.8%). The 35 patients with suspicious cervigrams were reevaluated colposcopically; 26 abnormal lesions were found and a directed biopsy specimen obtained. In 10 of the 26 patients, the histologic findings were negative for cervical neoplasia. In the other 16 patients there were three cases of CIN III, three cases of CIN II, and ten cases of CIN I. Of particular interest is the fact that one case of CIN III, two cases of CIN II, and six cases of CIN I were detected only by cervicography and had always had negative cytologic screening.

Tawa, from Kaiser Permanente of California, screened 3271 gynecology patients between the ages of 18 and 50 who had not had an abnormal smear in the last 6 months. The Pap smear and cervigram, both done during the same visit, were evaluated prospectively in a blind fashion. If the cervigram or Pap smear was positive, colposcopically directed biopsies were taken. There were 373 positive cervigrams and 39 positive smears. Seventy-two CIN lesions were detected by cervicography and 14 by Pap smears. Thus, 5.1 times the number of CIN lesions was detected by cervicography as compared with cytology. The cervigram was significantly more sensitive than the Pap smear, particularly for minor grade abnormalities. The Pap smear detected 14% of histologically proven CIN I, whereas the cervigram detected 88%. For CIN II, the Pap smear detected 38% of the cases, and the cervigram detected 85%.

Use

The place of this new technique in the practice of modern gynecology is still being discussed. Ideally, it should be used in conjunction with the routine Pap smear. Further research and evaluation are necessary to determine its cost effectiveness in this context. The method is of extreme value in follow-up of an abnormality detected by colpsocopy that does not require immediate therapy, documentation of the squamocolumnar junction prior to conservative ablation, especially if no endocervical curettage had been done, and training in colposcopy and research.

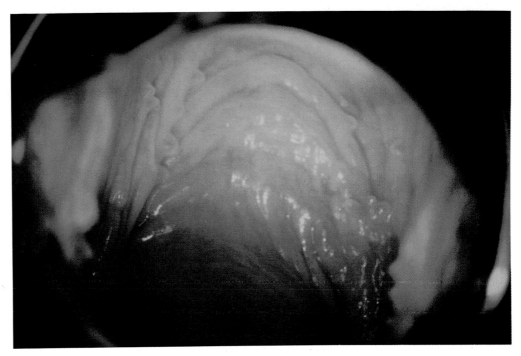

Color Plate 1. Anterior fornix of the vagina with normal squamous epithelium. Note the normal pink color.

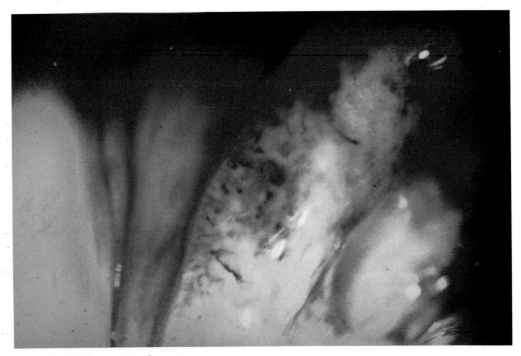

Color Plate 2. Side of the cervix with invasive squamous cell carcinoma. Note the nondividing atypical blood vessels.

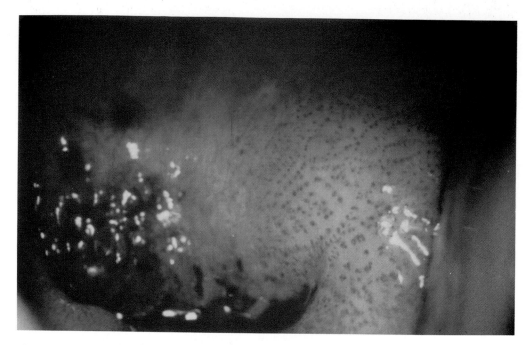

Color Plate 3. Cervix with cervicovaginitis secondary to trichomonas infection. Note the rosettes of punctate vessels without aceto-white epithelium.

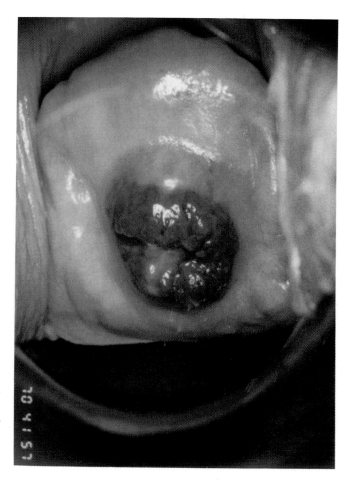

Color Plate 4. Healed cervix after laser vaporization. Note the columnar epithelium has a red appearance.

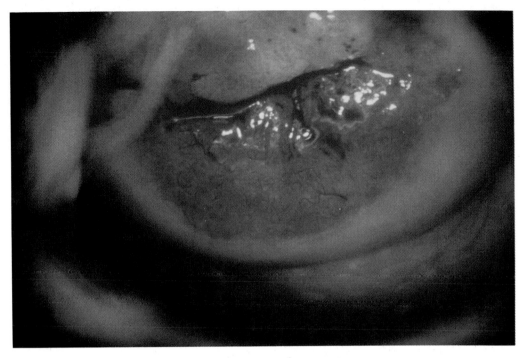

Color Plate 5. Cervix prior to acetic acid. Note the vascular change suggesting the presence of mosaic structure.

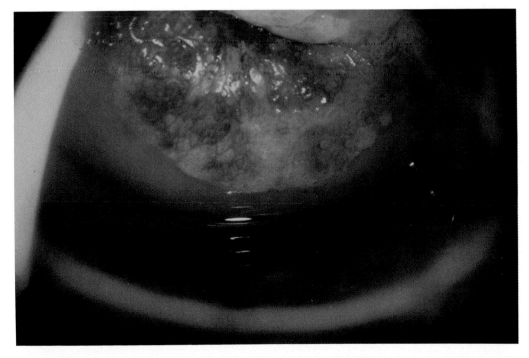

Color Plate 6. Cervix in Color Plate 5 after acetic acid. There is a grade II mosaic structure present. Biopsy revealed CIN II to III.

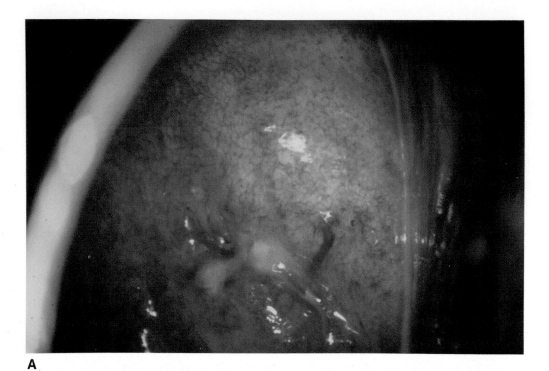

A

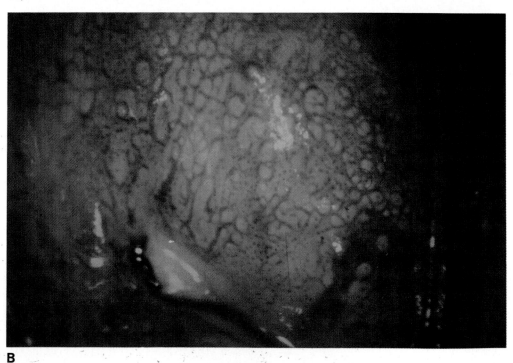

B

Color Plate 7. A. Cervix prior to acetic acid. Note the vascular arrangement suggesting a mosaic structure. **B.** Same cervix after acetic acid. There is an extensive mosaic structure present. Note that there are also areas of punctation intermingled with the blocks of mosaicism. Biopsy revealed CIN II.

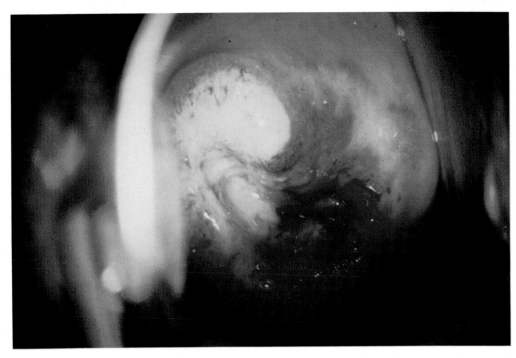

Color Plate 8. Cervix with invasive squamous cell carcinoma. Note the ulcerated posterior cervical lip. There is a raised white lesion on the side and anteriorly containing atypical blood vessels.

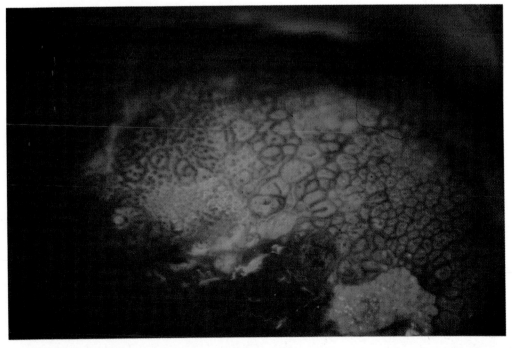

Color Plate 9. Anterior lip of the cervix after the application of acetic acid, showing punctation and mosaic structure.

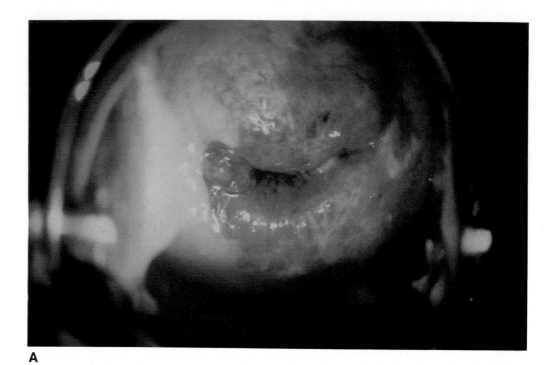

A

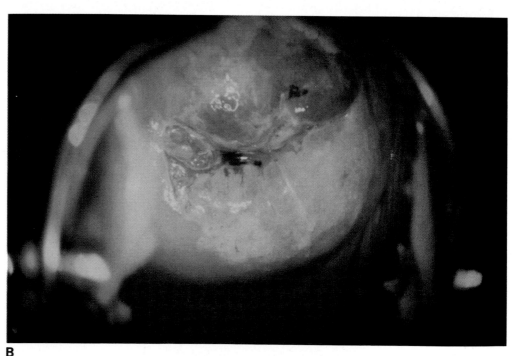

B

Color Plate 10. A. Cervix prior to acetic acid. The cervix looks innocuous. **B.** Cervix after acetic acid. Note the grade I aceto-white lesions on the posterior lip of the cervix from 3 to 7 o'clock.

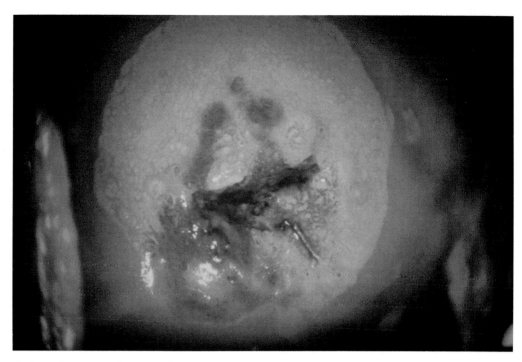

Color Plate 11. Cervix after acetic acid. There is a wide, atypical transformation zone in the form of a grade II mosaic structure. Biopsy diagnosed CIN II.

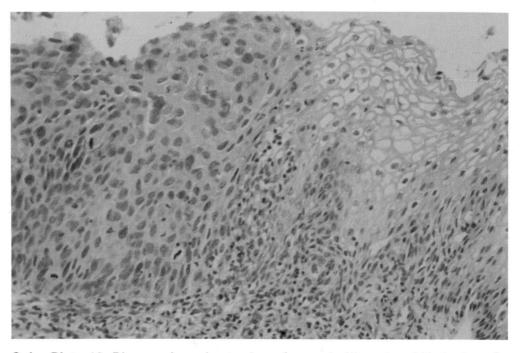

Color Plate 12. Biopsy of cervix at edge of a grade III aceto-white lesion. On the left side there is CIN II to III demarcated from an area of human papilloma virus.

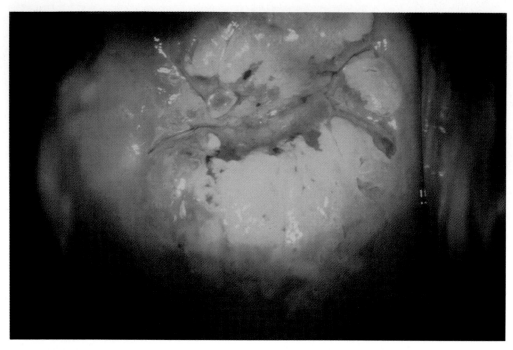

Color Plate 13. Cervix after acetic acid. The posterior lip has a raised, sharply delineated, grade III aceto-white lesion. Biopsy reported as CIN III.

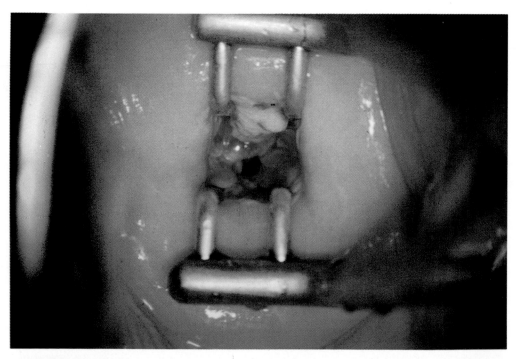

Color Plate 14. Colpophotograph of the endocervical canal being visualized with the aid of an endocervical speculum. An aceto-white lesion is on the anterior endocervical surface, extending almost to the internal cervical os.

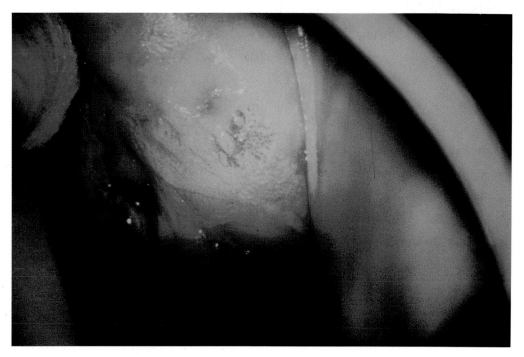

Color Plate 15. Cervix after the application of acetic acid. A cluster of atypical blood vessels stand out in a field of aceto-white epithelium at 9 o'clock.

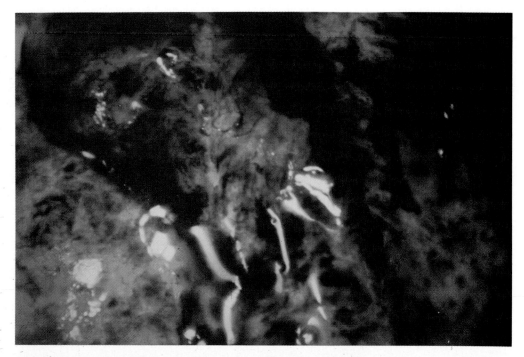

Color Plate 16. Cervix with invasive squamous cell carcinoma. Numerous atypical blood vessels are present; irregular in shape, parallel to the surface, nondividing, and friable.

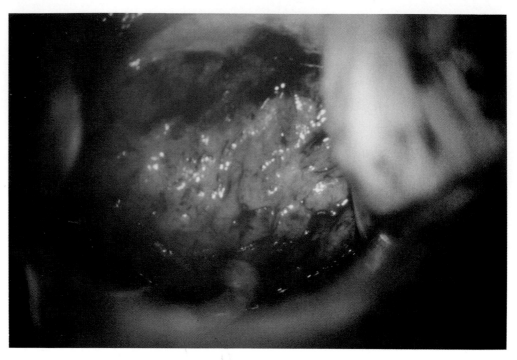

Color Plate 17. Posterior lip of cervix with invasive squamous cell carcinoma; note the yellowish hue as well as the abnormal blood vessels.

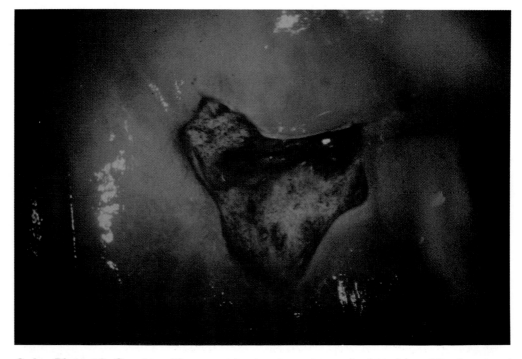

Color Plate 18. Cervix with a punched-out, endocervical lesion with abnormal blood vessels. Biopsy revealed adenocarcinoma.

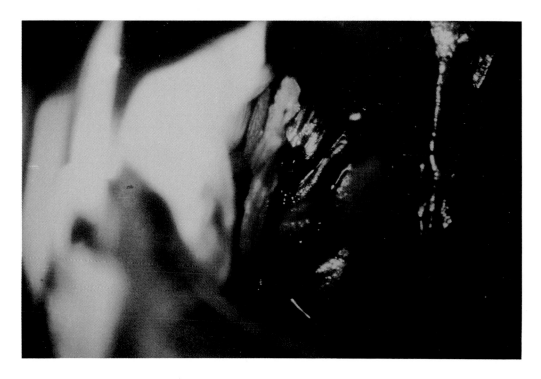

Color Plate 19. Vagina after Lugol's iodine stain. Note the raised, delineated, nonstaining areas that, on biopsy, showed VaIN III.

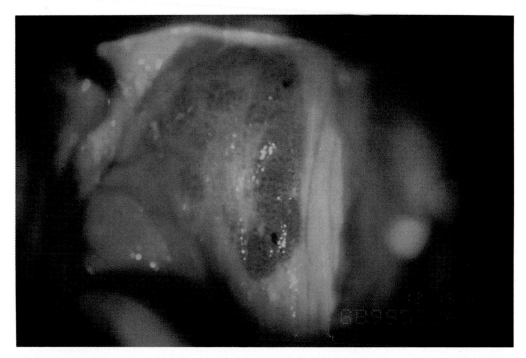

Color Plate 20. Apex of vagina before acetic acid. Note coarse punctation. Biopsy revealed VaIN III.

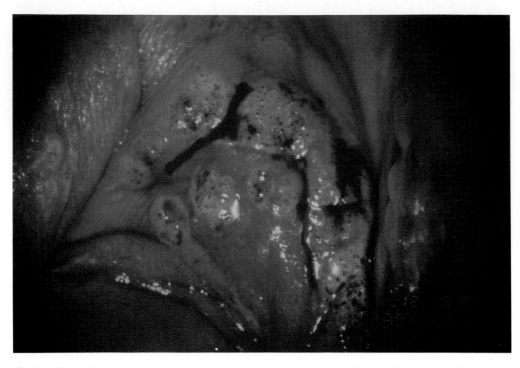

Color Plate 21. Apex of vagina showing coarse punctation with marked increase in intercapillary distances. Biopsy revealed early invasive carcinoma of the vagina.

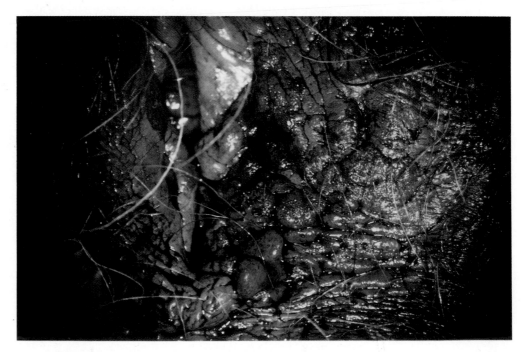

Color Plate 22. Vulvar lesion stained with 1% aqueous toluidine blue vital stain.

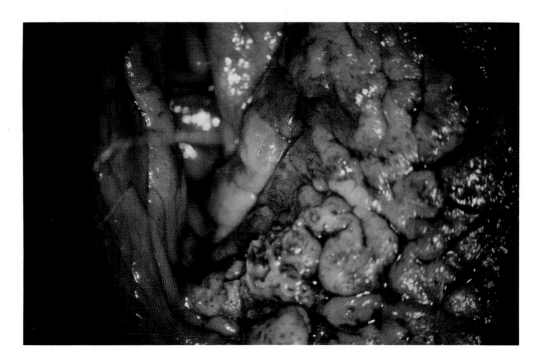

Color Plate 23. Lesion of Color Plate 22 after being washed with 1% acetic acid. Note areas of blue among the decolorized epithelium. Biopsy revealed VIN III.

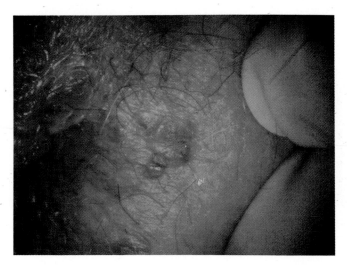

Color Plate 24. Lesion on the buttock treated with podophyllin. Note the absence of spicules and the flat appearance of the discoloration. Biopsy revealed VIN III.

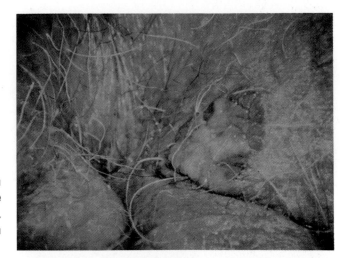

Color Plate 25. Lesion in the perianal area. Note the bluish discoloration. Biopsy is consistent with VIN III.

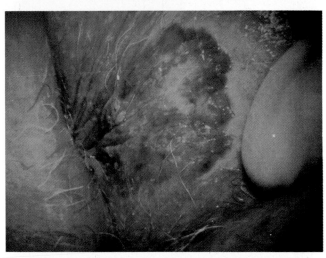

Color Plate 26. Variegated lesion on the perianal area. Biopsy revealed VIN III.

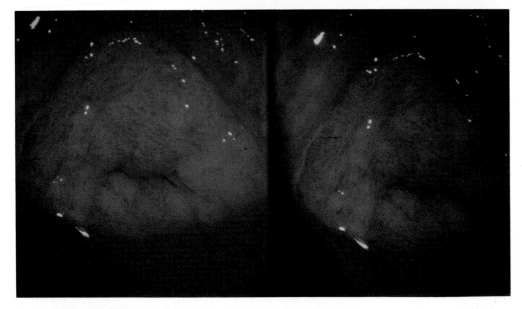

Color Plate 27. Cervix of a diethylstilbestrol exposed female before acetic acid. Note the red color due to the increased vascularity.

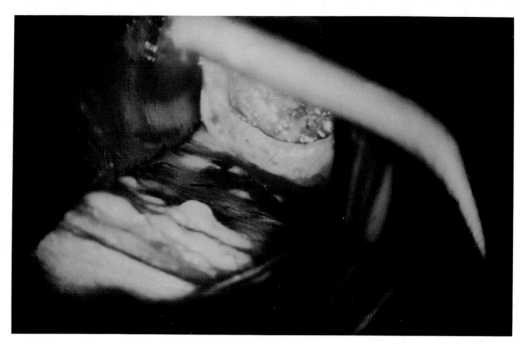

Color Plate 28. Diethylstilbestrol exposed patient with red nodular lesion (*arrow*) on the posterior vaginal wall. Biopsy showed clear cell adenocarcinoma.

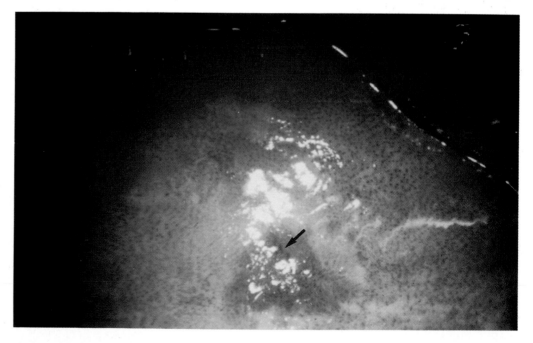

Color Plate 29. Nodule on the anterior vaginal wall of a diethylstilbestrol exposed female. Note the atypical blood vessels (*arrow*). Biopsy revealed clear cell adenocarcinoma.

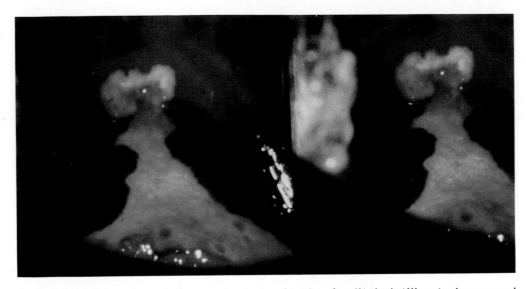

Color Plate 30. Iodine staining of anterior fornix of a diethylstilbestrol exposed patient. A triangular area of adenosis does not take the stain.

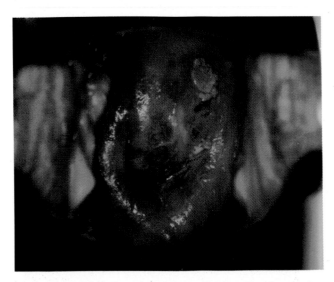

Color Plate 31. Atypical cervigram. Note the leukoplakia on the anterior lip of the cervix.

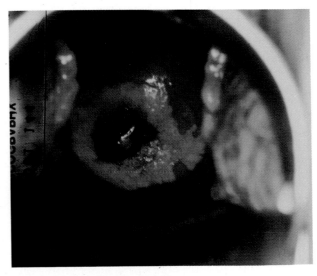

Color Plate 32. Positive cervigram with circumferential atypical transformation zone and the suggestion of a mosaic structure.

Bibliography

Abramson, AL, Steiberg BM, Winkler B. Laryngeal papillomatosis: Clinical histopathologic and molecular studies. *Laryngoscope*. 97:678–685, 1987.

Andersen, W, Frierson H, Barber S, et al. Sensitivity and specificity of endocervical curettage and the endocervical brush for the evaluation of the endocervical canal. *Am J Obstet Gynecol*. 159:702–707, 1988.

Anderson C, Hartley RB. Cervical crypt involvement by intraepithelial neoplasia. *Obstet Gynecol*. 55:546–550, 1980.

Anderson MC, Fraser AC. Adenocarcinoma of the uterine cervix: A clinical and pathological appraisal. *Brit J Obstet Gynaecol*. 83:320–325, 1979.

Andrews S, Hernandez E, Miyazawa K. Paired Papanicolaou smears in the evaluation of atypical squamous cells. *Obstet Gynecol*. 73:747–753, 1989.

Andrews S, Miyazawa K. The significance of a negative Papanicolaou smear with hyperkeratosis or parakeratosis. *Obstet Gynecol*. 73:751–753, 1989.

Antonioli DA, Burke L, Friedman EA. Natural history of diethylstilbestrol-associated genital lesions: Cervical ectopy and cervicovaginal hood. *Am J Obstet Gynecol*. 137:847–853, 1980.

Baggish MS. *Basic and Advanced Laser Surgery in Gynecology*. Norwalk, Conn: Appleton-Century-Crofts, 1985.

Baggish MS, Dorsey JH. Contact hysteroscopic evaluation of the endocervix as an adjunct to colposcopy. *Obstet Gynecol*. 60:107–110, 1982.

Ball HG, Berman ML. Management of primary vaginal carcinoma. *Gynecol Oncol*. 14:154–163, 1982.

Barron, SL. Sexual activity in girls under 16 years of age. *Br J Obstet Gynaecol*. 93:787–793, 1986.

Bearman, DM, MacMillan JP, Creasman WT. Papanicolaou smear history of patients developing cancer: An assessment of screening protocols. *Obstet Gynecol*. 69:151–155, 1987.

Benedet JL, Murphy KJ, Fairey RN. Primary invasive carcinoma of the vagina. *Obstet Gynecol*. 62:715–719, 1983.

Benedet JL, Sanders BH. Carcinoma in situ of the vagina. *Am J Obstet Gynecol*. 148:695–700, 1984.

Berek JS, Hacker NF, Fu YS, et al. Adenocarcinoma of the uterine cervix: Histologic variables. *Obstet Gynecol*. 65:46–52, 1985.

Bernstein SG, Kovacs BR, Townsend DE, et al. Vulvar carcinoma in situ. *Obstet Gynecol*. 61:304–307, 1983.

Bernstein SG, Voet RL, Gizick DS, et al. Prevalence of papillomavirus infection in colposcopically directed biopsy specimens in 1972 and 1982. *Am J Obstet Gynecol*. 151:577–581, 1985.

Bertani-Olivera AM, Kepler MM, Luisi A, et al. Comparative evaluation of abnormal cytology, colposcopy and histopathology in preclinical cervical malignancy during pregnancy. *Acta Cytol*. 26:636–643, 1982.

Bertrand M, Lickrish GM, Colgan TJ. The anatomic distribution of cervical adenocarcinoma in situ: Implications for treatment. *Am J Obstet Gynecol*. 157:21–25, 1987.

Betsill WL, Clark AH. Early endocervical glandular neoplasia: I. Histomorphology and cytomorphology. *Acta Cytol*. 30(2):115–126, 1986.

Boon M, Baak JP, Kurver PJ, et al. Adenocarcinoma in-situ of the cervix: An underdiagnosed lesion. *Cancer*. 48:768–773, 1982.

Bornstein J, Kaufman RH, Adam E, et al. Multicentric intraepithelial neoplasia involving the vulva: Clinical features and association with human papilloma virus and herpes simplex virus. *Cancer.* 62:1601–1604, 1988.

Bousfield L, Pacey F, Young Q, et al. Expanded cytologic criteria for the diagnosis of adenocarcinoma in-situ of the cervix and related lesions. *Acta Cytol.* 24:283–296, 1980.

Brescia RJ, Jenson B, Lancaster WD, et al. The role of human papillomaviruses in the pathogenesis and histologic classification of precancerous lesions of the cervix. *Human Pathol.* 17:552–559, 1986.

Broen EM, Ostergard DR. Toluidine blue and colposcopy for screening and delineating vulvar neoplasia. *Obstet Gynecol.* 38:775–778, 1971.

Brown LJ, Wells M. Cervical glandular atypia associated with squamous intraepithelial neoplasia: A premalignant lesion? *J Clin Pathol.* 39(1):22–28, 1986.

Brown MS, Philips GL. Management of the mildly abnormal Pap smear: A conservative approach. *Gynecol Oncol.* 22:149–153, 1985.

Burghardt E, Ostor A. Site and origin of squamous cell cancer: A histomorphologic study. *Obstet Gynecol.* 62:117–127, 1983.

Burke L. Diethylstilbestrol: Effect of in utero exposure. *Curr Prob Obstet Gynecol.* V(2):1–58, 1981.

Burke L, Antonioli, D. Vaginal adenosis. Factors influencing detection in a colposcopic examination. *Obstet Gynecol.* 48:413–421, 1976.

Burke L, Antonioli D, Friedman EA. Evolution of diethylstilbestrol-associated genital tract lesions. *Obstet Gynecol.* 57:79–84, 1981.

Burke L, Mathews B. *Colposcopy in Clinical Practice.* Philadelphia: F.A. Davis, 1977.

Buscema J, Stern JL, Woodruff JD. Early invasive carcinoma of the vulva. *Am J Obstet Gynecol.* 140:563–569, 1981.

Bychkov V, Rotman M, Bardawil WA. Immunocytochemical localization of carcinoembryonic antigen (CEA), alphafetoprotein (AFP), and human chorionic gonadotropin (HCG) in cervical neoplasia. *Am J Clin Pathol.* 79:414–420, 1983.

Caglar H, Hertzog RW, Hreshchyshyn MM. Topical 5-fluorouracil treatment of vaginal intraepithelial neoplasia. *Obstet Gynecol.* 58:580–583, 1981.

Campion MJ. Clinical manifestations and natural history of genital human papillomavirus infection. *Obstet Gynecol Clin N Am.* 14:363–388, 1987.

Campion MJ, Cusik J, McCance DJ, et al. Progressive potential of mild cervical atypia: Prospective cytological, colposcopic and virologic study. *Lancet.* 2:237–240, 1986.

Campion MJ, McCance DJ, Mitchell H, et al. Sublimeal penile human papillomavirus infections and neoplasia in consorts of women with cervical neoplasia. *Br J Genitourin Med.* 64:90–99, 1988.

Capen CV, Masterson BJ, Magrina JF, et al. Laser therapy of vaginal intraepithelial neoplasia. *Am J Obstet Gynecol.* 142:973–976, 1982.

Carson L, Twiggs LB, Fukushima M, et al. Human genital papilloma infections: An evaluation of immunologic competence in the genital neoplasia-papilloma sequence. *Am J Obstet Gynecol.* 155:784–789, 1986.

Choo YC, Hsu C, Ma H. The assessment of radioresponse of cervical carcinoma by colposcopy. *Gynecol Oncol.* 18:28–37, 1984.

Clarke EA, Hatcher J, McKeown-Eyssen GE, Lickerish GM. Cervical dysplasia: Association with sexual behavior, smoking, and oral contraceptives. *Am J Obstet Gynecol.* 151:612–616, 1985.

Conrad JT, Ueland K. Physical characteristics of the cervix. *Clin Obstet Gynecol.* 26:27–36, 1983.

Crippa L, DeVirgiliis G, Zoccoli A. Colposcopy in the postmenopausal period. Modification of mucosal atrophy by a short-term estriol treatment. *The Cervix & lfgt.* 5:143–219, 1987.

Crum CP, Egawa K, Fu YS, et al. Atypical immature metaplasia (AIM). A subset of human papillomavirus infections of the cervix. *Cancer.* 51:2214–2219, 1983.

Crum CP, Fu YS, Levine RU, et al. Intraepithelial squamous lesions of the vulva: Biologic and histologic criteria for the distinction of condylomas from vulvar intraepithelial neoplasia. *Am J Obstet Gynecol.* 144:77–83, 1982.

Crum CP, Levine RU. Human papillomavirus infection and cervical neoplasia: New perspectives. *Internl J Gynecol Pathol.* 3:376–388, 1984.

Daly JW, Ellis GF. Treatment of vaginal dysplasia and carcinoma in situ with topical 5-fluorouracil. *Obstet Gynecol.* 55:350–352, 1980.

Dotters DJ, Carney CN, Droegemueller W. Nylon brush improves collection of cytologic specimens. *Am J Obstet Gynecol.* 159:814–819, 1989.

Dunn JE, Crocker DW, Rube IF, et al. Cervical cancer occurrence in Memphis and Shelby County, Tennessee, during 25 years of its cervical screening program. *Am J Obstet Gynecol.* 150:861–864, 1984.

Ferenczy A. The biologic rationale for annual cervical cancer screening. *The Cervix & lfgt.* 3:25–31, 1985.

Ferenczy A, Mitao M, Magai N, et al. Latent papillomavirus and recurring genital warts. *N Eng J Med.* 313:784–788, 1985.

Fife KH, Rogers RE, Zwickl BW. Symptomatic and asymptomatic cervical infections with human papillomaviruses during pregnancy. *J Infect Dis.* 156:904–911, 1987.

Folkman J. Tumor angiogenesis: Therepeutic implications. *N Eng J Med.* 285:1182–1186, 1971.

Follen MM, Levine RU, Carillo E, et al. Colposcopic correlates of cervical papillomavirus infection. *Am J Obstet Gynecol.* 157:809–814, 1987.

Friedrich EG, Kalra PS. Serum levels of sex hormones in vulvar lichen sclerosus and the effect of topical testosterone. *N Eng J Med.* 310:488–491, 1984.

Friedrich EG, Wilkinson EJ, Fu YS. Carcinoma in situ of the vulva: A continuing challenge. *Am J Obstet Gynecol.* 136:830–843, 1980.

Fu Ys, Braun L, Shah KV, et al. Histologic, nuclear DNA, and human papillomavirus studies of cervical condylomas. *Cancer.* 52:1705–1711, 1983.

Fu YS, Lancaster WD, Richart RM, et al. Cervical papillomavirus infection in diethylstilbestrol-exposed progeny. *Obstet Gynecol.* 61:59–62, 1983.

Fu YS, Reagan FW, Fu AS, et al. Adenocarcinoma and mixed carcinoma of the uterine cervix: I. A clinicopathologic study. *Cancer.* 49:2560–2570, 1982.

Fu YS, Reagan JW, Fu AS, et al. Adenocarcinoma and mixed carcinoma of the uterine cervix: II. Prognostic value of nuclear DNA analysis. *Cancer.* 49:2571–2577, 1982.

Fu YS, Reagan JW, Richart RM. Precursors of cervical cancer. *Cancer Surveys.* 2:359–382, 1983.

Ghosh TK, Cera PJ. Transition of benign vaginal adenosis to clear cell carcinoma. *Obstet Gynecol.* 61:126–130, 1983.

Gilardi EM, Remotti G, DeVirgilis G, et al. Uterine cervix in pregnancy: I. Basic modifications and the dynamics of cervical mucosa. *The Cervix & lfgt.* 4:235–252, 1984.

Gloor E, Hurlimann J. Cervical intraepithelial glandular neoplasia (adenocarcinoma in-situ and glandular dysplasia). A correlative study of 23 cases with histologic grading, histochemical analysis of mucins, and immunohistochemical determination of the affinity for four lectins. *Cancer.* 58:1272–1280, 1986.

Goppinger A, Birmelin G, Ikenberg H, et al. Human papillomavirus standardization and DNA cytophotometry in cervical intraepithelial neoplasia. *J Reprod Med.* 32:609–613, 1987.

Hacker NF, Berek JS, Lagasse LD, et al. Carcinoma of the cervix associated with pregnancy. *Obstet Gynecol.* 59:735–746, 1982.

Hamou J, Salat-Baroux, J, Coupez F, et al. Microhysteroscopy: A new approach to the diagnosis of cervical intraepithelial neoplasia. *Obstet Gynecol.* 63:567–574, 1984.

Hannigan EV, Whitehouse HH, Atkinson WD, et al. Cone biopsy during pregnancy. *Obstet Gynecol.* 60:450–455, 1982.

Hatch KD, Shingleton HM, Orr JW, et al. Role of endocervical curettage in colposcopy. *Obstet Gynecol.* 65:403–408, 1985.

Hernandez-Linares W, Puthawala A, Nolan JF, et al. Carcinoma in situ of the vagina: Past and present management. *Obstet Gynecol.* 56:356–360, 1980.

Hoffman JS, Kumar NB, Morley GW. Microinvasive squamous carcinoma of the vulva: Search for a definition. *Obstet Gynecol.* 61:615–618, 1983.

Jaworski RC, Pacey NF, Greenberg ML, et al. The histologic diagnosis of adenocarcinoma in situ and related lesions of the cervix uteri. *Cancer.* 61:1171–1181, 1988.

Jones DED, Creasman WT, Dombroski RA, et al. Evaluation of the atypical Pap smear. *Am J Obstet Gynecol.* 157:544–549, 1987.

Jones RW. Malignant progression of carcinoma in situ of the cervix. *Colp Gynecol Las Surg.* 1:237–243, 1985.

Jordan JA, Singer A. *The Cervix.* Philadelphia: W.B. Saunders, 1976.

Kadish As, Burk PD, Kress Y, et al. Human papillomaviruses of different types in precancerous lesions of the uterine cervix: Histologic, immunocytochemical and ultrastructural studies. *Hum Pathol.* 17:384–392, 1986.

Kaminski PF, Norris HJ. Coexistence of ovarian neoplasms and endocervical adenocarcinoma.

Obstet Gynecol. 64:553–556, 1984.

Kaufman RH, Adam E, Noller K, et al. Upper genital tract changes and infertility in diethylstilbestrol-exposed women. *Am J Obstet Gynecol.* 154:1312–1318, 1986.

Kaufman RH, Korhonen MO, Strama T, et al. Development of clear cell adenocarcinoma in DES-exposed offspring under observation. *Obstet Gynecol.* 59:68s–72s, 1982.

Kishi Y, Inui S, Sakamoto Y, et al. Colposcopy for postmenopausal women. *Gynecol Oncol.* 20:62–70, 1985.

Kohan S, Beckman E, Bigelow B, et al. The role of colposcopy in the management of cervical intraepithelial neoplasia during pregnancy and postpartum. *J Reprod Med.* 25:735, 1980.

Kolstad P. The development of the vascular bed in tumours as seen in squamous-cell carcinoma of the cervix uteri. *Br J Radiol.* 38:216–223, 1965.

Koss LG. The Papanicolaou test for cervical cancer detection: A triumph and a tragedy. *JAMA.* 261:737–743, 1989.

Lacey CJN, Mulcahy FM, Sutton J. Koilocyte frequency and prevalence of cervical human papillomavirus infection. *Lancet.* 1:557–558, 1986.

LaPolla JP, O'Neill C, Wetrich D. Colposcopic management of abnormal cervical cytology in pregnancy. *J Reprod Med.* 33:301–306, 1988.

Lenehan PM, Meffe F, Lickrish GM. Vaginal intraepithelial neoplasia: Biologic aspects and management. *Obstet Gynecol.* 68:333–337, 1986.

Lozowski MS, Mishriki Y, Talebian F, et al. The combined use of cytology and colposcopy in enhancing diagnostic accuracy in preclinical lesions of the uterine cervix. *Acta Cytol.* 26:285–291, 1982.

Lunt R. Worldwide early detection of cervical cancer. *Obstet Gynecol.* 63:708–713, 1984.

McDonnell JM, Mylotte MJ, Gustafson RC, et al. Colposcopy in pregnancy. A twelve year review. *Br J Obstet Gynaecol.* 88:414–420, 1981.

McDonnell JM, Emens JM, Jordan JA. The congenital cervicovaginal transformation zone in young women exposed to diethylstilbestrol in utero. *Br J Obstet Gynaecol.* 91:574–579, 1984.

McIndoe WA, McLean M, Jones RW, et al. The invasive potential of carcinoma in situ of the cervix. *Obstet Gynecol.* 64:451–458, 1984.

McNab JCM, Walkinshaw SA, Cordiner JW, et al. Human papillomavirus in clinically and histologically normal tissue of patients with genital cancer. *N Eng J Med.* 315:1052–1058, 1986.

Meisels A, Fortin R. Condylomatous lesions of the cervix and vagina: I. Cytologic patterns. *Acta Cytol.* 20:505–509, 1976.

Meisels A, Morin C. Human papillomavirus and cancer of the uterine cervix. *Gynecol Oncol.* 12:111S, 1981.

Meisels A, Morin C, Casas-Codero M. Human papillomavirus infection of the uterine cervix. *Internat J Gynecol Pathol.* 1:75–79, 1982.

Melnick S, Cole P, Anderson D, et al. Rate and risks of diethylstilbestrol-related clear cell adenocarcinoma of the vagina and cervix. An update. *N Eng J Med.* 316:514–516, 1987.

Mene A, Buckley CH. Imvolvement of the vulval skin appendages by intraepithelial neoplasia. *Br J Obstet Gynaecol.* 92:634–638, 1985.

Merz B. DNA probes for papillomavirus strains readied for cervical cancer screening. *JAMA.* 260:2777, 1988.

Morrison BW, Erickson ER, Doshi N, et al. The significance of atypical cervical smears. *J Reprod Med.* 33:809–812, 1988.

Moseley KR, Tung VD, Hannigan EV, et al. Necessity for endocervical curettage in colposcopy. *Am J Obstet Gynecol.* 154:992–995, 1986.

Nasiell K, Roger V, Nasiell M. Behavior of mild cervical dysplasia during long-term follow-up. *Obstet Gynecol.* 67:665–669, 1986.

Nauth HF, Schilke E. Cytology of the exfoliative layer in normal and diseased vulvar skin. Correlation with histology. *Acta Cytol.* 26:269–283, 1981.

Noller KL. "DES-like" anomalies. *The Cervix & lfgt.* 3:285–288, 1985.

Noller KL, Stanhope CR. Colposcopic accuracy: Comparison of satisfactory examinations with results of conization. *Colp Gynecol Las Surg.* 1:181–184, 1984.

Noller KL, Townsend DE, Kaufman RH, et al. Maturation of vaginal and cervical epithelium in women exposed in utero to diethylstilbestrol (DESAD project). *Am J Obstet Gynecol.* 146:279–285, 1983.

Nuovo GJ, Blanco JS, Silverstein SJ, et al. Histologic correlates of papillomavirus infection of the vagina. *Obstet Gynecol.* 72:770–774, 1988.

Oliveira A, Keppler M, Luisi A, et al. Comparative evaluation of abnormal cytology, colposcopy and histopathology in preclinical cervical malignancy during pregnancy. *Acta Cytol.* 26:636–644, 1982.

Patterson JW, Kao GF, Graham JH, et al. Bowenoid papulosis. A clinicopathologic study with ultrastructural observations. *Cancer.* 57:823–836, 1986.

Peters WA III, Kumar NB, Morley G. Microinvasive carcinoma of the vagina: A distinct clinical entity? *Am J Obstet Gynecol.* 153:505–507, 1985.

Petrilli ES, Townsend DE, Morrow CP, et al. Vaginal intraepithelial neoplasia: Biologic aspects and the treatment with topical 5-fluoroucil and the carbon dioxide laser. *Am J Obstet Gynecol.* 138:321–328, 1980.

Purola EE, Halila H, Vesterinen E. Condyloma and cervical epithelial atypias in young women. *Gynecol Oncol.* 16:34–40, 1983.

Recher L, Srebnik E. Histopathologic features of koilocytotic atypia. A detailed description. *Acta Cytol.* 25:377–382, 1981.

Reid R. A rapid method for improving colposcopic accuracy. *Colp Gynecol Las Surg.* 3:139–146, 1987.

Reid R, Greenberg M, Jenson AB, et al. Sexually transmitted papillomavirus infection: I. The anatomic distribution and pathologic grade of neoplastic lesions associated with different viral types. *Am J Obstet Gynecol.* 156:212–222, 1987.

Reid R, Herschman BR, Crum CP, et al. Genital warts and cervical cancer: V. The tissue basis of colposcopic change. *Obstet Gynecol.* 149:293–303, 1984.

Reid R, Scalzi P. Genital warts and cervical cancer: VII. An improved colposcopic index for differentiating benign papillomaviral infections from high-grade cervical intraepithelial neoplasia. *Am J Obstet Gynecol.* 153:611–618, 1985.

Richart RM, Barron BA. Screening strategies for cervical cancer and cervical intraepithelial neoplasia. *Cancer.* 47:1176–1181, 1981.

Ridgley R, Hernandez E, Cruz C, et al. Abnormal Papanicolaou smears after earlier atypical smears with atypical squamous cells. *J Reprod Med.* 33:285–288, 1988.

Robboy SJ, Noller KL, O'Brien P, et al. Increased incidence of cervical and vaginal dysplasia in 3980 diethylstilbestrol-exposed young women. *JAMA.* 252:2974–2983, 1984.

Robboy SJ, Sugimura Y, Plapinger L, et al. Diethylstilbestrol and its consequences: Status in 1985. *The Cervix & lfgt.* 3:289–296, 1985.

Robboy SJ, Taguchi O, Cunha GR. Normal development of the human female reproductive tract and alterations resulting from experimental exposure to diethylstilbestrol. *Human Pathol.* 13:190–198, 1982.

Rome RM, Chanen W, Ostor AG. Preclinical cancer of the cervix: Diagnostic pitfalls. *Gynecol Oncol.* 22:302–312, 1985.

Rubio CA, Llatjos M. Kinetics of cell replication of the uterine cervix: IV. Proliferative loci in the basal cell layer. *Acta Cytol.* 26:367–369, 1982.

Sadeghi SB, Hsieh EW, Gunn SW. Prevalence of cervical intraepithelial neoplasia in sexually active teenagers and young adults. Results of data analysis of mass Papanicolaou screening of 796,337 women in the United States in 1981. *Am J Obstet Gynecol.* 148:726–729, 1984.

Saigo PE, Cain JM, Kim WS, et al. Prognostic factors in adenocarcinoma of the uterine cervix. *Cancer.* 57:1584–1593, 1986.

Sakuma T, Hasegawa T, Tsutsui F, et al. Quantitative analysis of the whiteness of the atypical cervical transformation zone. *J Reprod Med.* 30:773–776, 1985.

Salvaggi SM. Cytologic detection of condyloma and cervical intraepithelial neoplasia of the uterine cervix with histologic correlation. *Colp Gynecol Las Surg.* 3:115–123, 1987.

Sasson IM, Haley NJ, Wylander EL, et al. Cigarette smoking and neoplasia of the uterine cervix: Smoke constituents in cervical mucus. *N Eng J Med.* 312:315–316, 1985.

Schneider A, Sawada E, Gissman L, et al. Human papillomavirus in women with a history of abnormal Papanicolaou smears and in their male partners. *Obstet Gynecol.* 69:554–562, 1987.

Schneider A, Sterzik K, Buck G, et al. Colposcopy is superior to cytology for the detection of early genital human papillomavirus infection. *Obstet Gynecol.* 69:236–241, 1988.

Sedlacek TV, Cunnane M, Arpiniello V. Colposcopy in the diagnosis of penile condyloma. *Am J Obstet Gynecol.* 154:494–496, 1986.

Senekjian EK, Hubby M, Bell DA, et al. Clear cell adenocarcinoma (CCA) of the vagina and cervix in association with pregnancy. *Gynecol Oncol.* 24:207–219, 1986.

Shingleton HM, Gore H, Bradley D, et al. Adenocarcinoma of the cervix: I. Clinical evaluation and pathologic features. *Am J Obstet Gynecol.* 139:799–814, 1981.

Sillman F, Boyce J, Fuchter R. The significance of atypical vessels and neovascularization in cervical neoplasia. *Am J Obstet Gynecol.* 139:154–159, 1981.

Singer A, Wilters J, Walker P, et al. Comparison of prevalence of human papillomavirus antigen in biopsies from women with cervical intraepithelial neoplasia. *J Clin Pathol.* 38:855–857, 1985.

Soutter WP, Fenton DW, Gudgeon P, et al. Quantitative microcolpohysteroscopic assessment of the extent of endocervical involvement by cervical intraepithelial neoplasia. *Br J Obstet Gynaecol.* 91:712–715, 1984.

Soutter WP, Wisdom S, Brough AK, et al. Should patients with mild atypia in a cervical smear be referred for colposcopy? *Br J Obstet Gynaecol.* 93:70–74, 1986.

Spitzer M, Krumholz BA, Chernys AE, et al. Comparative utility of repeat Papanicolaou smears, cervicography and colposcopy in the evaluation of atypical Papanicolaou smears. *Obstet Gynecol.* 69:731–735, 1987.

Stafl A. Cervicograpy: A new method for cervical cancer detection. *Am J Obstet Gynecol.* 139:815–825, 1988.

Stafl A, Mattingly RF. Angiogenesis of cervical neoplasia. *Am J Obstet Gynecol.* 121:845–852, 1975.

Stenkvist B, Bergstrom R, Eklund G, et al. Papanicolaou smear screening and cervical cancer. What can you expect? *JAMA.* 252:1423–1426, 1984.

Syrjanen KJ. Female genital tract infections by human papillomavirus and their association with intraepithelial neoplasia and squamous cell carcinoma. *The Cervix & lfgt.* 2:103–126, 1984.

Tamimi HK, Figge DC. Adenocarcinoma of the uterine cervix. *Gynecol Oncol.* 13:335–344, 1982.

Tawa K, Forsythe A, Cove JK, et al. A comparison of the Pap smear and the cervigram: Sensitivity, specificity and cost analysis. *Obstet Gynecol.* 71:229–235, 1988.

Tay SJ, Jenkins D, Maddox P, et al. Subpopulation of Langerhans' cells in cervical neoplasia. *Br J Obstet Gynaecol.* 94:10–15, 1987.

Taylor PT, Andersen WA, Barber SR, et al. The screening Papanicolaou smear: Contribution of the endocervical brush. *Obstet Gynecol.* 70:734–737, 1987.

Teixeira WRG. Hymenal colposcopic examination in sexual offenses. *Am J For Med Pathol.* 2:209–215, 1982.

Toplis PJ, Casemore V, Hallam M, et al. Evaluation of colposcopy in the postmenopausal woman. *Br J Obstet Gynaecol.* 93:843–851, 1986.

Townsend DE, Levine RU, Crum CP, et al. Treatment of vaginal carcinoma in situ with the carbon dioxide laser. *Am J Obstet Gynecol.* 143:565–568, 1982.

Townsend DE, Richart RM, Marks E, et al. Invasive cancer following out-patient evaluation and therapy for cervical disease. *Obstet Gynecol.* 57:145–149, 1981.

Ulbright TM, Stehman FB, Roth IM, et al. Bowenoid dysplasia of the vulva. *Cancer.* 50:2910–2919, 1982.

Uldbjerg N, Ulmsten U, Ekman G. The ripening of the human uterine cervix in terms of connective tissue biochemistry. *Clin Obstet Gynecol.* 26:14–26, 1983.

van der Graaf Y, Vooijs GP. False-negative rate in cervical cytology. *J Clin Pathol.* 40:438–442, 1987.

van Nagell JR Jr, Greenwell N, Powell DF, et al. Microinvasive carcinoma of the cervix. *Am J Obstet Gynecol.* 145:981–991, 1983.

Walker PG, Singer A, Dyson JL, et al. Colposcopy in the diagnosis of papillomavirus infection of the uterine cervix. *Br J Obstet Gynaecol.* 90:1082–1086, 1983.

Watts KC, Campion MJ, Butler B, et al. Quantitative deoxyribonucleic acid analysis of patients with mild cervical atypia: A potentially malignant lesion? *Obstet Gynecol.* 70:205–207, 1987.

Weitrich D. An analysis of the factors involved in the colposcopic evaluation of 2194 patients with abnormal Papanicolaou smears. *Am J Obstet Gynecol.* 154:1339–1349, 1986.

Wells M, Brown LJR. Glandular lesions of the uterine cervix: The present state of our knowledge. *Histopathol.* 10:777–792, 1986.

Wespi HJ. Colposcopic-histologic correlations in the benign acanthotic nonglycogenated squamous epithelium of the uterine cervix. *Colp Gynecol Las Surg.* 2:147–158, 1986.

Wespi HJ. Enhancement of the colposcopic image of the uterine cervix by salicylic alcohol and metacresol-sulphonic acid. *The Cervix & lfgt.* 4:139–148, 1986.

Wilczynski SP, Walker J, Liao SY, et al. Adenocarcinoma of the cervix associated with human papillomavirus. *Cancer*. 62:1331–1336, 1988.

Wilkinson EJ, Rico MJ, Pierson KK. Microinvasive carcinoma of the vulva. *Intnl J Gynecol Pathol*. 1:29–39, 1982.

Woodling BA, Hegar A. The use of the colposcope in the diagnosis of sexual abuse in the pediatric age group. *Child Abuse Negl*. 10:111–114, 1986.

Woodman CBJ, Jordan JA, Wade-Evans T. The management of vaginal intraepithelial neoplasia after hysterectomy. *Br J Obstet Gynaecol*. 49:707–711, 1984.

Zinser HK, Rosenbauer KA. Untersuchungen uber die angioarchitecktonik der normalen und patholigisch veranderten cervix uteri. *Achiv Fur Gynakol*. 194:79–112, 1960.

Zunzonegui MV, King MC, Coria CF, et al. Male influences on cervical cancer risk. *Am J Epidem*. 123:302–307, 1986.

Zur Hausen H, Gissman L, Schlochofer JR. Viruses in the etiology of human genital cancer. *Prog Med Virol*. 30:170–188, 1985.

Index

Page numbers followed by f refer to figures and by
t to tables. Color plates are indicated by CP followed
by the figure number.